THE
REAL
MAN'S
TOOL BOX

THE

REAL

MAN'S

TOOL BOX

A DIY HEALTH MANUAL FOR MEN

TAMMY FARRELL

IMPORTANT NOTE TO READERS: Although every effort has been made to ensure the contents of this book are accurate, it must not be treated as a substitute for qualified medical advice. Always consult a qualified medical practitioner. Neither the author nor the publisher can be held responsible for any loss or claim arising out of the use, or misuse, of the suggestions made or failure to take advice.

hachette
AUSTRALIA

Published in Australia and New Zealand in 2009
by Hachette Australia
(an imprint of Hachette Australia Pty Limited)
Level 17, 207 Kent Street, Sydney NSW 2000
www.hachette.com.au

National Library of Australia
Cataloguing-in-Publication data:

Farrell, Tammy.

Real Man's Tool Box / Tammy Farrell.

9780733623943 (pbk.)

Men--Health and hygiene.
          Health behavior.
          Health attitudes.

613.04234

Cover and internal design by Christabella Designs
Illustrations throughout by Bob Shields; i-bobshields.blogspot.com
Typeset in Berkeley by Pindar NZ, Auckland

Hachette Australia's policy is to use papers that are natural, renewable and recyclable products and made from wood grown in sustainable forests. The logging and manufacturing processes are expected to conform to the environmental regulations of the country of origin.

To Mum, Dad, Scott, Mark, Michelle & to my dearest nanna who passed during the beginning stages of this book – thank you for all your unconditional love, support & encouragement.

Contents

Introduction

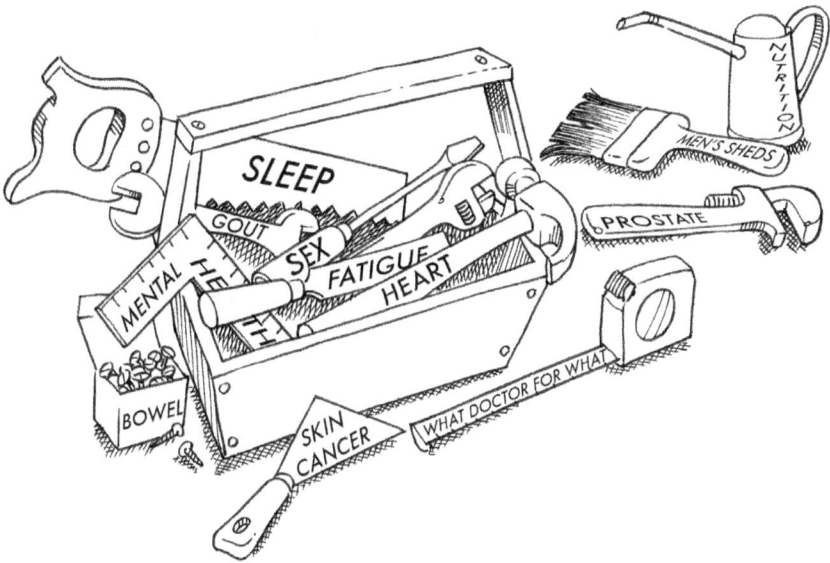

Maybe you use your body to run or play cricket or golf. Maybe you just use it to sit on the beanbag and open a tinnie, or to light the barbie and watch the missus turn the snags. Maybe you used to be a surfer and now you're just a couch surfer.

Whichever use you put your body to, it's a safe bet that you never think too hard about how it works . . . until it doesn't.

I hope you're reading this book before the wheel falls off the axle, but it's likely that you're reading it because you have to – your wife or mother or sister or doctor has probably forced you to read it.

Well, good. I've got you now. And I plan to tell you as much as possible about your body in as short a space as possible, so you can get back to whatever it is you were doing before you started reading . . . But, hopefully, *not* back to your bad habits.

WAIT!

I'm not saying you have to give up the tinnies, the red wine, or even the snags. (But you'll definitely have to give up the fags.) All you need to do is read and pay attention, and also realise that most of what you fear need never happen to you, provided you take care of a few simple things.

Still with me?

You may have noticed that I'm not actually a bloke, which may cause you to wonder why you should pay any attention to what I have to say to you. It's true – I have XX chromosomes. What's also true is that I have a *lot* of experience talking about everyday health in the workplace, mainly to coalminers and blokes who work in largely XY-dominant companies. I first had the idea to develop this type of service when I worked as a registered nurse in an Intensive Care Unit and would often receive calls from my two brothers – both working as tradesmen – asking health-related questions for either themselves or their workmates.

As years passed and I was still answering questions, I came up with a question of my own: why do men take their car to the mechanic as soon as there's even a little rattle, but they run in the other direction from a doctor when they need to look under their own hood? So I asked some blokes I've known since I was a kid what they knew about their bodies – what they actually knew about what is and isn't normal about their bodies. They all laughed and said, 'That's what you're here for, Tam – you can tell us!' Hmmm . . .

While it's all very well for my brothers and their mates to ask me questions, I realised that lots of Aussie blokes may not have an on-call nurse to turn to when something is niggling them. And something *always* niggles eventually.

This book is my way of being unofficially on-call for all of you – and, really, you all need the help. I'm not talking about muscle strains and compound fractures, either. This book is mainly about the subterranean stuff: your gut and your bowel, your heart and your, um, *bits*. It's also about how you're sleeping, how you're performing in the bedroom (are there things you want to change but don't know the right person to ask how?) or as you younger blokes like to call it 'shagging' and whether you need to get a shed. Because I've realised that most of you *will* go to a doctor if one of your panels is dented, but not if your radiator is leaking. And which one do you think is more important for keeping the metaphorical car on the road?

There's also a little bit of information to help you understand the women in your lives – don't get too worried, there won't be anything too gruesome. Just the stuff you need to know in order to make life easier for you and them. Given that your significant female other – whether she's related to you or sharing your bed – is the first, if not only, person you're likely to consult when you have a health problem, it's only fair that you know something about what might make life harder for her from time to time. That's not too much to ask, is it?

You may not want, or need, to read this book from cover to cover, although I'd obviously like you to. You can just read the chapters you need when you need them, and that's okay. Just make sure you read them – that's all I ask. I haven't written this for my own amusement – if that was my motivation, I'd just keep taking calls from my brothers and the rest of the crew.

Each of us wants to have a happy, healthy life, even when we appear to be working towards the opposite end. And as prevention is really the best form of cure, it stands to reason that learning more about how to keep your bits healthy *before* they go downhill is a sure-fire way to keep life sweet. That's really why I'm writing this: to keep you on the golf course or on the Board or at the track – all right, if you must – in the beanbag or sitting in that favourite armchair. It's what I want for all the blokes in my life – and now that includes you.

Tammy Farrell
2009

A healthy ticker: your human heart

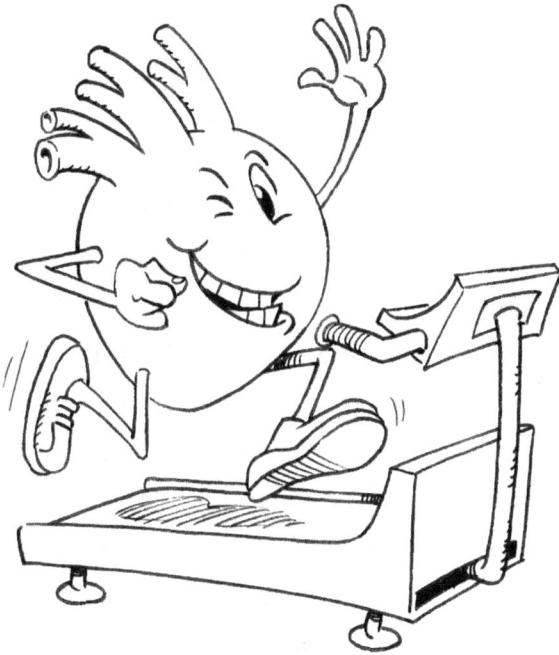

Everyone's got one. Most people have no idea how it works until it goes wrong, but they'll blame it for all sorts of decisions: 'I was listening to my heart, not my head'; 'Bloody ticker, keeps playin' up on me'; and, most commonly from dads to their daughters, 'What is it love? A broken heart, get rid of the idiot, he was nothin' but a pain in the a—'

Come on, you know you've done it. But do you even know what your heart looks like? Do you know exactly how it functions, apart from 'Well, I think it keeps me alive'? Shame on you! It's time you learnt, because heart disease is Australia's biggest killer, and it's a bugger of a way to die. One in two Aussie men run the risk of developing heart disease, and I'm not just talking about heart attacks, either. The really silly thing is that in most cases it's preventable.

Pull up the beanbag and get comfy – there's a bit to learn in this chapter.

The parts

Most of us know that the heart sits in the top part of our torso, a little bit to the left. What you may not know is that it's made up of four chambers.

The chambers allow blood to enter from the top right-hand side of the heart into the right atrium, through a valve (tricuspid) to the bottom chamber (right ventricle) through another valve (pulmonary semilunar) into the lungs to exchange some carbon dioxide for some oxygen, back into the left side of the heart to the top chamber (left atrium), through another valve (bicuspid) to the left ventricle on the bottom, then out through the last valve (aortic semilunar) to the aorta moving blood away from the heart to the rest of the body and to your brain. It's probably easier to remember the letter A for AWAY: the aorta pumps blood *away* from the heart.

I haven't lost you yet have I? Keep reading, it will make sense . . . I'll give you the short version in case you're reading this while watching *The Footy Show*. There will then be a long version for those of you whose wives are watching *Desperate Housewives*.

The heart works as a complex pump. So it can work effectively it requires its own :
- Plumbing system or blood supply to the heart muscle as fuel; and
- Electrical system coordinating the pump's activity.

Basically the heart is like a car engine all on its lonesome, and all in one convenient small size. Now, read on, but it does get technical.

Pumping is the Key

The heart is actually a muscle, and it works as a pump to keep blood flowing throughout the body. Each time your heart beats, blood is being pumped around the body – this is what you hear when you listen to your pulse. (This may sound like commonsense to you, but some people do not realise that . . . so please don't think I'm being condescending, I just want to make sure you are following).

The heart is positioned directly behind the sternum, a long bone which connects to our ribs. If you're doing CPR, it's the sternum you press on, and this act of compression pumps blood around the body and, most importantly, to the brain.

Sorting out the plumbing

The heart has its own plumbing system supplying blood to the heart muscle.

Try to visualise your arteries – your really important blood vessels – as long pipes. There are three main coronary arteries –

the blood vessels going to your heart: the left anterior descending artery, circumflex artery and right coronary artery. They're like the plumbing built around the foundation of a house. These arteries service various areas of the heart. Just as your house pipes drain away waste products – to and from the bathroom, laundry or kitchen – keeping your house running smoothly, the arteries keep your heart supplied with only the good stuff: oxygenated blood. Without oxygenated blood, the heart muscle doesn't work.

Coronary arteries are tiny but they have a huge responsibility. If the coronary arteries become blocked or narrowed due to cholesterol or a plaque build-up, the blood supply to that specific part of the heart will be constricted or stopped, potentially causing a great deal of pain. This episode is technically known as a myocardial infarction or, more commonly, a heart attack. It means heart muscle death – and once the heart muscle is dead that part of the muscle will not rejuvenate itself . . . once its dead, it's dead!

You may know or be someone who had a stent implanted after a heart attack. A stent is a metal coil inserted into the diseased artery which helps to hold the artery open. Or maybe you or your mate have gone the next step and had the blocked coronary artery bypassed in surgery, using a vein to do a similar job. It's unlikely that you'll go through life without someone you know having a stent or a bypass – but wouldn't it be great if they didn't? Wouldn't it be great if *you* didn't? Prevention is always better than cure. Look after your heart!

Fiddling with the electrics

The heart has its own electrical system, triggering impulses for each heartbeat. In order for all the four chambers of our heart to work together, electrical impulses constantly and consistently trigger the heart to beat in sequence, starting from the top of the heart in the atria, following an electrical path down to the bottom of the heart to the ventricles. In a healthy human being the heart beats anywhere from 86 400 to 144 000 times per day And that's while they're relaxing. That's a lot! No wonder we need to sleep at night.

In the medical world we call this path of electrical impulses the 'conduction system'. The conduction system consists of spark plugs, otherwise known as 'nodes'. Each node has its own important role, starting with the sinoatrial node at the very top of the sequence, the atrioventricular node, his bundle, right and left bundle branches, and finally the conduction myofibres. I am sure this all makes sense if you're handy with the electrical side of life.

If one of these spark plugs is not working properly it will affect the whole conduction system – you may have a very fast pulse even when you're just sitting reading a book, or you may have a very slow pulse which causes you to fall over or feel dizzy, or even have irregular beats affecting your daily life.

These types of problems can be fixed through medication or medical procedures, so see your doctor if you're concerned.

The upkeep

Blood pressure

Blood pressure (BP) is, unsurprisingly, the pressure of the blood in your arteries as it is pumped around the body by the heart. When the heart pumps, blood in the arteries rises and falls in a regular 'wave' pattern. BP peaks when the heart pumps – this is called systole, which represents the top number in a BP reading. It falls when the heart relaxes – this is diastole, which represents the bottom number.

Normal blood pressure is considered to be around 120/80 mmHg (this represents the measurement in millimetres of Mercury, as was used in the day of a mercury filled pressure measuring device) – so the systole is 120 and the diastole is 80.

Your blood pressure can never relax to 0, unless you're dead. A residual amount of blood is always sitting in the heart, like oil in an engine, keeping the motor (and the BP) ticking over. Of course, once it runs dry it's all over for the motor.

Why measure blood pressure?

Let's treat BP as if it's tyre pressure. In order to know if you've got enough air in your tyres, you need to go to the servo and wait for the bloke in the Torana to finish checking his Goodyears, and then you clip on the hose and find out whether you need to pump them up or not. And just because they're fine this week doesn't mean that they'll be fine in four weeks' time, after you've taken your precious beast on the Sofala road then around Mount Panorama as you daydream about Lowndes and Whincup. In fact, if you had done this you probably wouldn't even wait to get back to Sydney before checking your tyres – you'd probably do it in Bathurst when you fill up the tank. So why would you assume that your blood pressure at the age of fifty-four – after many years of unpaved roads and high-speed tracks – would be the same as it was at twenty-four?

I often ask blokes why they make sure they have enough pressure in their truck or car tyres, and the answer is always quite logical: 'It's for better performance and handling, better traction – and it's safer'. Well, my point exactly . . .

So you need to measure your BP so you know just how hard your heart is working and, accordingly, whether you need to do something about it. Ideally you should have your BP checked at least once a year, during a visit to your GP (you know, the doctor you're meant to see every once in a while?).

However, if you have a personal or family history of high blood pressure, stroke or heart attack, you should have it checked a little more frequently. Even if you're not worried about your BP, ask your doctor to tell you what it is next time you're having a check-up. It's a fun fact to know, and it also helps you get an idea of where you're sitting on the scale of things.

If you develop some kind of blood pressure fetish or legit-imately need to check your BP on a regular basis, you can buy your own BP machine from most chemists.

High blood pressure

High blood pressure is also referred to as hypertension. It's one of the greatest risk factors for heart disease, stroke, heart failure and kidney disease. The good news is that you can fix it. Medication can help and you can also try to eliminate some of the risk factors mentioned below.

To help you rank your blood pressure, here's a handy scale –

note that high BP is considered to be anything over 140/90 mmHg:

Normal – 120/80 mmHg
Stage 1 – 140/90 mmHg
Stage 2 – 160/100 mmHg
Stage 3 – > 180/110 mmHg

Risk factors for high blood pressure

If even one of the following applies to you, you'll need to keep an eye on your BP.

- You have a family history of high BP.
- You're a smoker.
- You're overweight or obese.
- You're regularly in stressful situations.
- Your alcohol consumption is heavy.
- You eat a diet high in salt.
- You have diabetes.

I can't tell you how often I see slender patients coming in to the clinic saying, 'But I couldn't have high blood pressure – I'm thin. Only fat fellas have high blood pressure'. Bad news; it's not just the overweight who have high BP. I also hear overweight people telling me that they're 'fit and healthy because my blood pressure is within normal limits'. This is also no cause for celebration – it simply means that their heart has learnt to compensate for the added blood vessels and tissue it must supply with blood, but nine times out of ten their pulse will be beating out of control and their lungs will also be hard at work.

Reasons to not have high blood pressure

Think of your heart as being like a body builder – like Ah-nuld Schwarzenegger in his Conan days. As body builders get bigger, their muscles get less flexible – they look impressively strong but they probably can't even tie their own shoelaces.

The same applies to the heart; the higher your blood pressure, the harder your heart muscle works, thickening this part of the muscle and causing it to tire easily. Soon it doesn't have the ability to squeeze the ventricle together in order to eject enough blood around the body. The end result is heart failure. Then there are other cheerful outcomes like stroke, brain haemorrhage and heart attack.

So the moral of this story is: don't be Ah-nuld.

Moreover, if you eat badly enough you'll end up with fatty plaque in your blood vessels. And if you have fatty plaque plus high BP, well . . . consider yourself to be the proud owner of a three-lane highway that has suddenly had two lanes blocked, and all the cars on the road now have to move into one. (I'm sure you've been in that situation, and you know how bloody long it takes to merge.) The walls of your arteries will stage their own little road-rage incident and you'll end up with a stroke or a heart attack. And the moral of *this* story is: three lanes really don't merge into one without someone blowing a gasket.

The big worry is if there's a narrowing of your carotid artery, which is located in your neck (don't worry, you can't nick it while shaving) and supplies blood to your brain. It's a bit like trying to blow up a balloon while pinching off the end – not a lot of air gets in and it takes a helluva long time for the balloon to inflate. That balloon is your brain. And it's hard to have a party with a saggy old balloon.

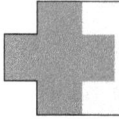

The 50 000 Km service

We've already established that the heart has a lot of work to do. In fact, it works more than most organs in the body – it starts beating when you're a foetus, and that's before you have a brain and well before you need to use your lungs. And like anything that works hard, it's prone to wearing out, particularly if you don't take care of it.

Which is all a roundabout way of saying that there is a lot that can go wrong with your heart. For some of it you can blame your relatives and the DNA they gave you; for most of it you can blame yourself. But before you do, let's have a little look at some of these potential problems – all the better to head them off at the pass, eh?

Atherosclerosis

As atherosclerosis is the underlying cause of a lot of heart disease, it's worth a closer look. In fact, the most common cause of heart disease is a decrease in blood supply as a result of atherosclerosis, so it's kind of important that you know about it.

Atherosclerosis is the name for lipid- or fat-rich deposits a.k.a. plaque (not the same kind that's on your teeth and which your dentist should be scraping off for you – because you're going to the dentist regularly, right?). The plaque lines the inside walls of your blood vessels. It's often caused by high cholesterol in our blood. And while you can have an inherited tendency to have high cholesterol, it's definitely something that can be controlled by what you eat.

Atherosclerosis remains undetected until the plaque becomes large enough to impair the blood flow to a blood vessel. In most cases symptoms don't really show up until there's a blockage of more than 70 per cent of one or more coronary arteries in most people who have it.

So what?

I'll give it to you straight: atherosclerosis causes angina and can certainly lead to a heart attack. A heart attack can kill you, as I'm sure you know. The best way to prevent the heart attack is to not get atherosclerosis.

Atherosclerosis is when an artery has become blocked due to plaque or coronary spasms. Often plaque is quite toxic to the blood vessel, and this causes the blood vessel to collapse and appear extremely tight.

When this narrowing of the artery reduces blood flow to the heart, it also causes you intense pain when having a heart attack. The heart's literally being starved of oxygenated blood. If it's starved for too long, the heart muscle dies. This doesn't happen suddenly – atherosclerosis develops over time so you may now be paying for the damage you started doing in your younger years. But making changes to your habits will make a difference so don't think it is too late.

Risky business

The risk factors for developing heart disease are similar to those for high blood pressure, which shouldn't really be a surprise. The number one risk factor is your parents – I mean, if your parents had heart disease. One parent bad; two parents extra bad.

Other risk factors include:
- Your sex: heart disease is more common in males than females (they catch up after menopause).
- High blood pressure.
- Foods high in saturated and trans fat.
- Hypertension.
- Smoking.
- Diabetes.
- Eating processed foods and foods high in sugar.
- Heavy alcohol consumption.
- Stressful personality/environment.
- Obesity.
- Lack of physical activity.

If you've read other chapters in the book you may have noticed that a lot of these risk factors are the same as for other serious illnesses. You may also have noticed that there's a really common theme: diet and exercise. If you eat fat, you get fat. If you don't do anything to burn off that excess fat, it's even worse. Seriously, eating chips and drinking a whole lot of soft drink just isn't worth the drama of heart disease. You don't have to give them up – just don't have them every day. And move your arse off the couch. You're built for speed and power – your body is made for running and lifting. Lifting a remote control and running after the paper boy just won't do it.

Son of atherosclerosis: cardiovascular disease

Cardiovascular disease is, in truth, heart, stroke and blood vessel disease. It often occurs as a result of atherosclerosis. Cardiovascular disease can be seen in the legs, carotids (blood vessels located in the neck) or any areas where there are blood vessels. So, pretty much everywhere.

The other son of atherosclerosis: coronary heart disease

This is what happens when the coronary arteries become clogged or blocked with fat deposits, otherwise known as plaque. The affected arteries narrow, limiting the amount of blood that can flow down them. Because these arteries supply your heart with oxygen, less blood flow means less oxygen.

If the heart isn't receiving as much blood as it should, it will be under greater stress. The heart is not an organ that gets a lot of downtime, so it doesn't really have the capacity for a lot more stress on a regular basis. Consequently, if it's asked to work harder – such as during exercise or walking up stairs – you may start to experience difficulties. These difficulties will likely manifest as chest pain, angina or even a heart attack.

So when you hear the term 'Ischaemic Heart disease' it simply refers to the lack of blood supply to an area of the heart. It is also the number one killer of Australians.

Angina versus heart attack

Angina is temporary chest discomfort or pain, and it doesn't last very long – a few minutes. Angina doesn't damage your heart, and it will resolve itself when you rest or take anginine spray, which allows the arteries to relax to normal.

A heart attack is more severe, and if the artery remains blocked for a significant amount of time, the heart is then permanently damaged. The pain of a heart attack can be excruciating, but there is also such a thing as a 'silent' heart attack, when the sufferer may feel only slight discomfort, and it's only confirmed later, through blood tests, that the person suffered a heart attack.

The technical name for a heart attack is myocardial infarction or MI.

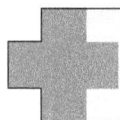

The 150 000 Km service

Let's talk a bit more about heart attacks because far too many people get them and don't know anything about them until they have one. Believe me, you'd rather not have one, and knowing a bit more about them could help you prevent one.

Heart attacks usually occur in people over forty-five years of age. Anyone at that stage of life is probably going to have a lot on – job, family, friends, hobbies – so they could be forgiven for not noticing the first signs of a heart attack. Because heart attacks can progress over several hours, they can be hard to detect at first. It pays to know your body well so that you can pick up these early signs in the midst of your noisy life. But if you don't know your body that well, just be alert to progressive changes that could signal the development of something serious.

You're more at risk of a heart attack if you:

- Smoke.
- Have a family history of heart disease and/or heart attacks – if your siblings, mother or father have had heart problems, it is highly likely you too will experience problems at a similar age.
- Are a diabetic.

- Have high cholesterol.
- Use recreational drugs.

Now, you may think I put in that last item because all medical professionals have a 'just say no' attitude to drug use. And it's true, we do – mainly because of what we see at work.

It's not true, though, that drugs are only a bad risk if you're buying them from a dodgy dealer. My first problem with that is: how do you know if the dealer's dodgy? And if you know beforehand that the dealer's dodgy, why buy drugs from them? I've seen too many young, socially active people die or almost die from using drugs they thought were okay because they only bought the 'good, expensive stuff'.

I once cared for a 21-year-old who had a massive heart attack after using cocaine all night. Earlier he had smoked joints with friends, then the group of twenty or so moved onto cocaine while celebrating a friend's birthday. My patient was on the floor for twenty minutes before a friend went over to see what was going on. Initially the friend admitted he had seen him on the floor ten minutes earlier and, thinking he had passed out, chose to leave him there. A further ten minutes went by and the friend decided maybe something was wrong. When three friends knelt down to wake the patient they tried to find a pulse; it was so fast they couldn't count it.

At this point their mate's heart was in ventricular fibrillation (VF) – it was pounding so fast it was out of control. Consequently his heart didn't have time to fill with blood in order to pump blood to the rest of the body, let alone his brain. Bad news for him. For approximately twenty-seven minutes this young guy received very little blood to his brain. If his friends had even commenced CPR, they could have helped get some more blood to his brain, but paralysed by the fear of not knowing what was going on; they were unable to do anything.

At least they rang an ambulance – unlike some idiots who, in a similar situation, wouldn't call the ambulance because they think they'll get arrested for drug possession. The ambos aren't cops – keep that in mind.

This young man was in intensive care for six weeks on a ventilator, being given medications to keep his heart pumping properly. Once he was weaned off the medications and could breathe for himself he left our unit. He had to learn to walk again, eat by himself and re-learn the basics of life. He had severe memory loss, but was fortunate to have the love and guidance of a very loving family to help him deal with the long-term effects.

No doubt he never thought that, at twenty-one, he'd have a heart attack. But he did and it could happen at any age.

What to look out for

If you or someone you're with starts to show the following symptoms, call an ambulance.

- Pain, although a silent heart attack can occur in the elderly and in diabetic people (20 per cent of cases).
- A crushing, tight feeling; some describe it as heaviness in the chest.
- Pain radiating from the neck, throat, jaw, shoulders, back, both arms, wrists and hands
- Possibly nausea and vomiting.
- Shortness of breath.
- They appear extremely fatigued with a lot of sweating, and a drop in blood pressure will cause the person to look pale, feel clammy and almost ready to faint.

- If you feel their pulse, bear in mind that a normal pulse should be between 60 to 100 beats per minute. If it's higher than this and the person is at rest, something's not right.

It's important to know that in the case of both angina and a heart attack, the sufferer won't feel pain in the heart itself. We have no pain receptors in the heart – they are located around the heart, hence a heart attack affects the nerves in the shoulder blade which shoot down to your little finger, and the nerves around the chest area or to the jaw. This is why sometimes people do think it's only 'indigestion'.

> **Remember:** a heart attack will not cause pain in the heart itself. Don't ignore the symptoms above, thinking you're not having a heart attack unless the heart itself hurts.

Want to hear something strange and kind of ridiculous? A 2007 survey by the Heart Foundation found that 56 per cent of people in New South Wales would not call an ambulance when experiencing heart attack signs or symptoms. Some of them said they'd rather phone a friend than waste an ambulance's time if it wasn't really anything serious.

I'm here to tell you that a heart attack is not *Who Wants to be a Millionaire*. Unless your friend is a cardiologist, all they can help you with are sympathetic noises while your life ebbs away. If you're a taxpayer – especially one with health insurance – then you're perfectly entitled to call an ambulance or go to casualty for chest pain. If it turns out to be nothing, the ambos won't get cross at you. They'd be more cross if they got there too late to do anything because you were too busy asking a friend whether your chest pain was option A, B, C or D.

CASE STUDY

I recall meeting one 43-year-old gentleman in the hospital at three o'clock on a Sunday morning. He had been rushed into the emergency department with chest pain. This man told us he'd had chest pain since 11 a.m. on the Saturday, but had had a barbecue to go to with his wife, and he was playing poker with the boys at 7 p.m. He didn't want to ruin his plans and make a fuss, so he ignored the niggling feeling during the day. Once he arrived at poker he thought a good strong scotch might fix it, while puffing on his token cigar. At this point he still hadn't mentioned it to anyone.

He arrived home at 11 p.m., telling his wife that he wasn't feeling the best. By 1 a.m. he confessed he had chest pain and told his wife, 'I think I'm having a heart attack. There's a lot of pressure in my chest.'

The gentleman had a 95 per cent blockage to one of his major coronary arteries; he was very lucky he made it to us alive. He didn't believe a 43-year-old could have a heart attack, so he'd put it down to his own imagination.

This gentleman was fortunate because he lived only ten minutes away from a large Sydney training hospital. Medical help was easily at hand, with an angioplasty clinic only three levels away. If you live further away from medical help – especially if you're in the country – you do not have the time to sit back and hope the pain goes away.

If this situation happens to you, tell somebody and call an ambulance. You won't be making a fuss! And who cares if you are, anyway? It's better than ending up dead.

Stop it before it starts

Of course, if you're really concerned about making a fuss, stop the heart attack before it even starts. Prevention is always much less fuss than cure. If you have one or more of the risk factors mentioned above – particularly if heart disease is in your family – you should change the following lifestyle factors slowly and in a realistic manner.

These lifestyle factors will, by now, sound familiar.

1. Quit smoking. I actually can't believe I have to say this, but some of you insist on lighting up.
2. Aim to reach your ideal body weight. Ask your doctor to tell you what that is – don't try to guess.
3. Get some regular exercise, but this doesn't mean getting on a rowing machine. Simply walking each day is a great way to keep your heart healthy; and it really is best to start any exercise program slowly.
4. Control your blood pressure, even if that means just taking your BP medications routinely. It may also mean learning to keep your stress at manageable levels.
5. If you're diabetic, keep it under control.

Don't be one of those people who waits for a heart attack to be their 'wake-up call' – unless you're some kind of magician, you won't get to decide whether your heart attack is fatal or not, so you really won't know if you'll wake up or not. I do get cross when I see people not taking care of their health, heading straight for a heart attack, because ignoring your health can have such an impact on people's lives. Next time you think your love of bad food and inactivity is more important than anything else, think of your wife or kids having to spoon-feed you because your clogged arteries gave you a heart attack so massive that you end up in a wheelchair. Or maybe you won't even get to see your kids grow up because, despite the fact your dad had a heart attack at fifty, you keep smoking a pack a day. I don't understand how your ciggies or your hamburgers or your ten hours a day in front of the television is actually worth that outcome. If you'd like to explain it to me, go ahead – but I've yet to find anyone who can.

The really, REALLY important thing I want you to remember is that heart attack-proofing your life doesn't mean that you're making it boring. You don't have to exercise every day. You don't have to give up your favourite foods. You just have to learn how to be moderate in everything.

Except cigarettes. They really have to go. And think twice about your recreational drug use – it may seem like a reasonably priced high at the time, but a few months in hospital is expensive.

SOME USEFUL CONTACTS
- www.heartfoundation.com.au
- www.heartfoundation.org.au

The mysterious world of the prostate

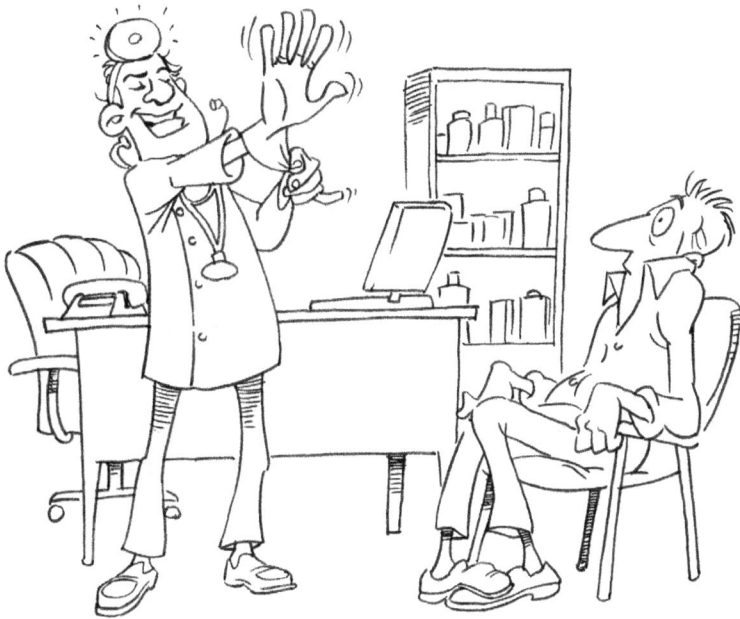

The parts

If you have a prostate, then you're the member of an exclusive club: Man-world. Yes, that's right – only blokes have prostates. And let's make sure we pronounce it correctly: pros-TATE. Not to be confused with pros-TRATE, which is what you do in a Catholic church as you approach the altar, or how you find yourself when you've had a few too many shandies and not enough food.

Normally the prostate is no bigger than a walnut, and it sits just below the bladder. The urethra – the tube carrying urine and semen out through the penis – runs through the prostate. If your prostate becomes enlarged you'll find you have difficulty urinating – the enlarged prostate presses down on the urethra, partially blocking the flow and putting pressure on the bladder. Not at all comfortable, and not unlike what happens to women when they're pregnant, only in that instance there's a whole baby putting pressure on the bladder.

The prostate is surrounded by many blood vessels, nerves and muscles required to:

1. maintain normal bladder control;

2. aid an erection.

I know this bloke called Paul Scarfe, who's a prostate cancer survivor (there's a bit about Paul later). He likes to compare the prostate to the airconditioning in a car: 'The car will still function well without one but it's a luxury few men would choose to do without'. And that would be because the prostate's main role is to produce most of the fluid in semen.

I had to giggle one day when a rather hefty patient with a gruff-sounding voice told me he had initially come to hospital due to his 'tubes . . . you know . . . me fallopian tubes, I think'. He was actually referring to his prostate and urethra, but I told him I was impressed that he knew fallopian tubes existed. If you have no idea what I'm talking about, read the 'Secret Women's Business' chapter.

How does it work?

Before ejaculation takes place, the prostate gland squeezes a mucous-like fluid through your urethra in order to mix with the sperm and further mucous. It then sits in the seminal vesicle.

You're probably wondering why our body bothers with extra fluid if it's not all sperm, right? Like everything in the human body, there's a purpose to it, and that is to protect the sperm by keeping it in an alkaline (non-acidic) environment, which helps it stay alive so it can (if you're lucky) enter inside the vagina and potentially fertilise an egg. It may come as a shock to you to discover that *every* act of sexual intercourse is designed to create babies but that is, in fact, the case and you may choose to remember this at the point at which you decide that a condom is too much trouble . . .

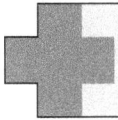

The 50 000 Km service

It's considered normal for a prostate to grow in size as you start to age, but this growth is dependent on the hormone testosterone, which is produced in the testes. If there's a problem with the testosterone levels, you may also get problems with the prostate.

There's a handful of conditions that can affect the prostate, and it's worth going through them in a bit of detail because they may happen to you or someone you know – and forewarned is forearmed.

Prostatitis

Prostatitis is inflammation of the prostate gland. (As a point of curiosity, 'itis' attached to anything means 'inflammation of'.)

Prostatitis is not overly common. It can be either a short- or long-term problem, but it's certainly not considered to be life threatening. You may hear it being referred to as acute prostatitis or chronic prostatitis.

Acute prostatitis is not very common, but when it happens it most commonly affects those between the ages of twenty-five and fifty. It is caused by a bacterial infection which creates inflammation around the gland, making it quite tender. The symptoms are similar to that of a bladder infection, with pain on urination, pain on ejaculation, pain within the anus and the scrotum, along with possible chills and fever.

Chronic prostatitis is also caused by a bacterial infection. The inflammation tends to be longer lasting, arising after an episode of acute prostatitis or for no particular reason at all. The symptoms are similar to that of the acute prostatitis but the individual may also experience pain towards the lower abdomen and the shaft of the penis, radiating to the testes and inner thigh.

Enlarged prostate

An enlarged prostate does not automatically mean you have something dire; it's also referred to as a 'benign prostate enlargement' or a 'benign prostate hyperplasia'. This is quite common among our older generation.

Many of the fellas I have dealt with in the hospital environment have admitted that as soon as they started having problems 'piddling', they expected the worst and cancer came into their minds straightaway – a few of them said they figured that if they ignored it, it might just go away. Yeah . . . that never ends so well, does it? I can't think of a single medical condition that gets better when it's ignored. Can you?

If the following symptoms sound familiar, please don't think they'll just go away. They won't!

- Wanting to urinate frequently throughout the night while lying down (which puts further pressure on the bladder).
- You may feel that the need to urinate becomes 'urgent'.
- There's a sensation of wanting to urinate but when you start, nothing comes out – not only is this quite frustrating, but the sensation doesn't dissipate.
- Uncontrolled leaking or dribbling after going to the toilet.

If these symptoms make you suspect you may have a prostate problem, see your local GP. You may then have two possible tests.

- The prostate specific antigen (PSA) blood test.
- Digital rectal examination (DRE).

The 150 000 km service

The most serious prostate condition you can develop is cancer. Approximately 18 700 Aussie men were diagnosed with prostate cancer in 2006; 3000 men die as a result of prostate cancer each year. One in five men will have prostate cancer by the age of eighty-five; it's the most common cancer diagnosed in Australia (excluding non-melanoma skin cancers) and the second largest cause of male deaths related to cancer.

Prostate cancer is considered to be quite a slow-growing form of cancer, developing when cells in the prostate start to grow at a faster pace than considered normal, forming a malignant tumour.

Prostate cancer cells break away from the prostate as the tumour gets bigger, causing harm to the bones and lymph nodes in the neighbourhood, potentially causing more tumours, which we refer to as metastases. It's best to detect this cancer before it spreads any further.

According to Cancer Council Australia, the prospect of developing prostate cancer increases due to factors such as:

- family history – if your father or brother has had prostate cancer you have three times the risk of other blokes;
- age – the older you are, the higher the risk.

In the early stages of prostate cancer, you often won't see or feel symptoms. This is obviously a concern, hence the reason medical professionals urge you to have your PSA levels checked from the age of fifty or, if you have a positive family history, from the age of forty.

The symptoms

The symptoms common in those with advanced prostate cancer may vary but most commonly they are:

- Blood in urine or semen.
- Pain during urination.
- An urgency or need to urinate.
- Difficulty when trying to urinate.
- Having to urinate too often.
- Pain around the thighs and hips.

These symptoms can be caused by other health problems, but if you have them you should make an appointment with your doc sooner rather than later. It may be nothing. If it's cancer, though, speed is your friend. You're not going to be able to change the fact that it's cancer – especially by ignoring the symptoms – but if you can get a diagnosis as early as possible, it will improve your chances of a good outcome.

Here's a little cautionary tale – read it to make sure you get the message.

CASE STUDY

I'm fit, I jog, cycle and lead an active lifestyle. Four years ago my dad (aged seventy-two) went to see his doctor due to constantly having 'to take a pee'. 'Old man syndrome', we all thought. But the doctor was confident he had prostate cancer and scheduled him for a biopsy; he also told him that his sons should be checked, and we all dutifully were.

Just a jab and stab (a vulgar term I've coined) – that is, a blood test and a finger up the bum (in layman's terms). Not something the average bloke wants to dwell on but no big deal in reality. To cut a long story short: my dad and both my older and younger brothers results were clear of cancer but I had it.

How the hell could I have cancer!? I look after myself, I don't smoke, I eat correctly, I'm not overweight, I exercise – crikey, I had just run a half marathon up Mt Wellington. Nope they've messed up the result with my dad's, I thought. Several tests later confirmed that I definitely had cancer and my PSA was increasing. I did my research and elected for surgery. Today I'm cancer-free and leading the same lifestyle as before. No continence or impotence problems of any significance and the future's so bright I have to wear shades.

Many of us spend too much of our efforts investing in our wealth and precious little investing in our health; without your health, wealth is futile. My advice is to get tested before you turn fifty, and invest in a healthy lifestyle. I know there are blokes out there thinking it won't happen to them, like the smokers who candidly say, 'You have to die from something'. Well, try mixing with a few terminal cancer sufferers like I did and you'll get a whole new perspective about this precious gift of life, that we all too often take for granted!

Paul Scarfe, prostate cancer survivor

The tests

The prostate specific antigen (antigen refers to a level of protein or level of antibodies in the blood made by the cells, which has the ability to cause an immune response) – otherwise known as the PSA or prick test – is a blood test looking for the level of protein (antibodies) made by the cells in both a normal and a cancerous prostate. Due to the natural enlargement of the prostate as you age, it's normal to have a slow rise in PSA levels, but it is also important to be aware, as the Cancer Council Australia highlights, that 'only one in three men with an elevated PSA level will have cancer'. This test is certainly not the ultimate diagnostic tool as it is just a marker – it needs to be used in combination with the other tests, such as a digital rectal exam and a biopsy.

In terms of numbers you may hear your doctor tell you, a PSA reading of 10 is considered high and would put you in the 'at risk' category but this is something you should chat about with your GP to make sure you understand what the different levels mean.

The PSA level is also useful if you are diagnosed with cancer, as it can be used to monitor the growth of the prostate and the effectiveness of the cancer treatment. The higher the PSA level rises, the greater the rate of cancer growth.

A digital rectal examination (DRE) sounds unpleasant but it is an effective tool, allowing a doctor to feel for any enlargement or hardening of the prostate gland. This test involves the doctor inserting his or her finger (gloved, of course) into your rectum to feel for the prostate. He or she is feeling for a hardening of the prostate or an abnormal enlargement. Or both.

I once met a patient who was obviously feeling extremely uncomfortable and self-conscious about having a rectal examination but seemed to deal with everything through humour. When the doctor had his finger in the patient's rectum the doctor said, 'No, there doesn't seem to be any enlarged areas', the patient asked, 'Would you mind using your second finger?' The doctor paused, and the patient finished by saying, 'I want a second opinion . . .' The doctor was speechless, not used to someone joking at this delicate moment!

The rectal exam *can* be uncomfortable, but it shouldn't be painful. It should be used in combination with the PSA level test as it is not 100 per cent effective due to the doctor only having access to a portion of the prostate because of the confined space within the rectum.

A biopsy is performed if you have had a positive finding (hardening or enlarged areas) on your rectal examination and/ or you have high levels of PSA on your blood test. The biopsy allows the urologist – the specialist – to take a specimen of the tissue in suspicious areas within the prostate. The tissue is sent to a pathologist for further testing to confirm whether there are cancerous cells present. If cancer cells are present, the pathologist will be able to analyse what grade and what stage the cancer is.

In order for the urologist to detect the suspect area, an ultrasound-like camera known as a trans-rectal ultrasound (try saying that three times fast) is used. This is a probe containing an ultrasound generator accompanied by sampling needles. It's inserted into the rectum, allowing the medical team to see relatively clear pictures of the prostate. The vision on the monitor allows the doctor to see where exactly they need to insert the sampling needles in order to obtain a specimen. And you'd really need to have some kind of fetish to enjoy it, so I'm not even going to try to tell you to lie back and relax. Just grit your teeth and bear it. Of course, there's sedation or anaesthesia for your comfort, and the procedure is usually performed in a day clinic so it won't take too much time out of your life.

The Gleason score is a grading system for any cancer cells found. They are graded according to their severity, from low risk to highly aggressive. Please refer to the chart below.

Gleason score	Aggressiveness of prostate cancer
2–4	Low
5–6	Moderate
7	Intermediate
8–10	High

Source: *Prostate Cancer Foundation of Australia*

According to the Prostate Cancer Foundation of Australia, 'a score of 2 to 5 indicates the cancer is relatively slow-growing and possibly not very aggressive. A score from 5 to 7 indicates the cancer is faster growing and moderately aggressive. A score of 8 or higher indicates an aggressive cancer.' Don't try to decipher things yourself. Ask your doctor and keep asking questions until you understand.

Prostate cancer is, unfortunately, one of those things we rarely hear about unless it becomes fatal. Often it's not talked about because men feel too embarrassed to discuss it, or they have ongoing symptoms for years and don't want to cause a fuss so don't bother getting it seen to unless it really starts to give them grief. Things may be changing, though – the radio/television personalities such as Alan Jones and AFL commentator Sam Newman have recently been diagnosed with prostate cancer and have publicly discussed their experiences. There really is nothing to be embarrassed about – cancer is a disease and if it happens to you, you won't be the only person you know with cancer. Just because it's in your prostate doesn't mean you can't talk about it.

Let's just look at this one last time, so you can minimise your chances of prostate cancer adversely affecting your life.

1. Get tested regularly if you are the age of fifty or over.
2. If there is a family history, get tested from the age of forty.
3. If you have symptoms, please see your doctor no matter what age you are.

And here's a nifty motto to help you remember:
'You know the trick: go get the prick.'

SOME USEFUL CONTACTS

- www.prostate.org.au

The bowel does what?

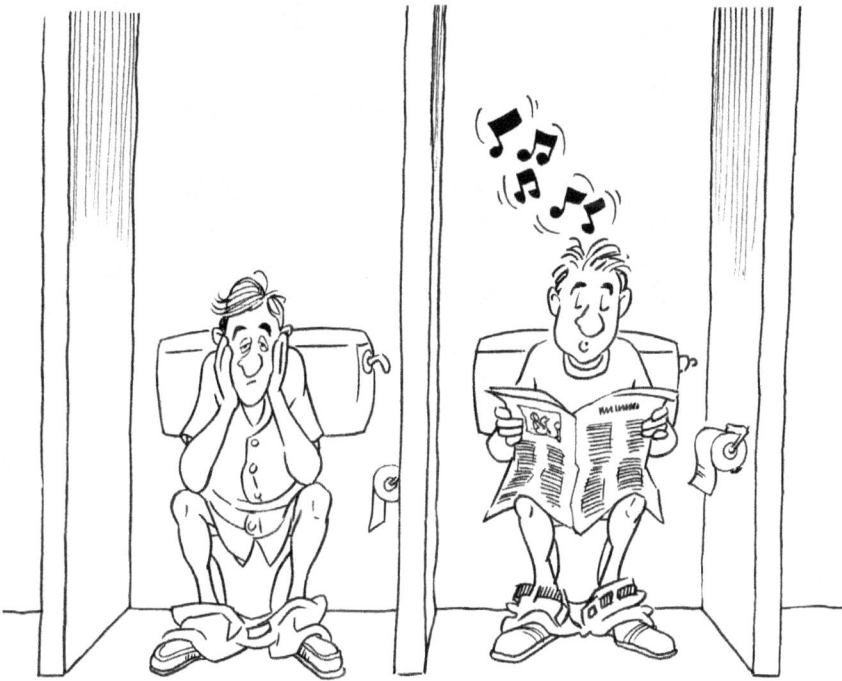

Regardless of our age, nationality, sex or social status, there is one thing that unites us as human beings. We all poo. Although we have lots of different names for it: shit, crap, dump, etc, it all means the same thing. In fact, 'poo' should be the verb used to teach English grammar in primary school: *I poo, you poo, we poo*. Because it's true – we do.

So we all poo – but how much do you know about your poop chute? Do you even know that it's called the BOWEL?

Well, now you do.

You should also know that most people's bowels will keep on keepin' on – with the odd interruption, like diarrhoea – until they drop dead. But some people's bowels won't. And for some the bowel can be like a footy game. Some people's bowels will play fast and loose, or they'll block a tackle every single time. You may be one of those people. In the most unfortunate of cases, you will be the person whose bowel is sent to the sin bin permanently. And wouldn't you rather not get sent off?

I'm of the mindset that prevention is better than the cure in *all* cases, especially when it's so easy to take care of the prevention part. There's a lot you can do to prevent most of the nasty stuff, and not all of it involves eating bran cereal.

It's possible that you're reading this chapter because you think you've retired from the game: you have bowel cancer. That's clearly a rotten gig. But it doesn't mean you can never get back on the field, so there's some info here for you too.

Okay, no bran cereals! I promise (but they actually aren't that bad!).

Let's get the hard data out of the way first.
- Percentage of people who poo: 100 (as we already know this, you can skip this line).
- Number of Australians diagnosed with bowel cancer each year: 4000.
- Number of Aussie blokes who will have bowel cancer by the age of eighty-five: 1 in 10 (and don't presume you won't live until eighty-five . . . those doctors are trying to keep us

alive until we're 150 so the Rudd Bank can get more GST out of us).

- Number of cases of bowel cancer that can be cured if detected early enough: 9 out of 10.

In short, the bad news: the older you get, the more likely it is you'll get bowel cancer. And the good news: early detection gets results.

Here's what you need to know about early detection.

1. Know what your poo usually looks like. (Doctors like to call poo 'stools' but I always think there's a danger of miscommunication here especially in a hospital setting when the doctor asks 'would you pass me the stool please' . . . 'I meant a seat . . .' 'Oh'.
2. Know your family history. If a close relative – male or female – has had bowel cancer then you'll need to have regular checks.
3. If you have no family or previous personal bowel cancer history and you're over the age of fifty, you'll need to have a regular screening test.
4. If your poo looks significantly different over a period of time – bearing in mind the fact that beetroot always has an alarming affect on poo – then bite the bullet and go to the doctor. YES, THE DOCTOR.

Here's another thing, you need to know about early detection: quite often, what you're detecting isn't anything sinister. Poo is such a regular and easily accessed tracker of your health – it helps you measure the function of your stomach, liver, intestines and bowel – that it's no wonder early physicians used it as a diagnostic tool for all sorts of ailments.

So it makes sense to keep track of your poo – especially when smelling it is not a requirement. Taking a peek in the toilet bowl doesn't mean you're weird. Looking at your poo is the most painless check you can do and just means you're taking advantage of your body's very natural processes to monitor your own wellbeing. And you don't need to leave the house to do it!

Don't take my word for it though. Here's a story you need to read.

CASE STUDY

Imagine experiencing diarrhoea for three months, not wanting to say anything in case you're overreacting. Slowly the diarrhoea – five to eight times per day – becomes a little more urgent, to the point where you start a bit of a trot on your way to the bathroom. Before you know it, you've shifted your bedside lamp into the bathroom.

Five days into the emergency bowel motions, you look down and there is now fresh blood: sometimes clots, sometimes not . . . This happened to someone I know.

'Dave', as I'll call him, went to his GP and was referred to a gastroenterologist – a gut and bowel specialist – and within days he had an appointment. Dave had had polyps several years earlier. They'd been removed, and he'd been instructed by the doctor at the time to come back every two years for a check-up to minimise the risk of developing further complications, such as more polyps and – worst case – bowel cancer.

Dave, now sixty-six years of age, had missed four check-ups – almost ten years' worth – and the receptionist who took the patient profile he filled in at the specialist's rooms was clearly disapproving when she looked over the details. This didn't make Dave feel any better – and nor did the sight of a man who walked out of the doctor's office looking very drawn and pale, and being rushed off for an emergency endoscopy – that's the procedure where they stick a thing up your . . . Actually, I don't think I need to explain that now.

The doctor booked Dave in for a colonoscopy (commonly referred to as the 'silver stallion' by many blokes – and if you take care of yourself properly you need never find out why) and a gastroscopy (a camera stuck down your throat to check out the stomach and small bowel).

The tests revealed that Dave had three polyps of considerable size and a haemorrhoid, which was causing the bleeding. So it wasn't cancer – but it could have been. And if only he'd had his regular check-ups he could have avoided the diarrhoea and the bleeding and the silver stallion.

I'm not even trying to be subtle here: there's just no substitute for taking care of things. You put your car in for service; you put wax on your surfboard, you even get your golf clubs cleaned. When did your car and your clubs become more important than *you*? You certainly can't surf when you're dead, no matter which soft-focus view of the afterlife you have.

But I can huff and puff all I like, and I still won't make an impression if I can't explain to you exactly *why* it's so important to take care of your bowel. So I think the best thing is to tell you a bit more about it. After all, you're carrying one around every second of your life – it's time you made friends with it.

The parts

The bowel is a V8 Commodore of an organ (that's enough, Ford lovers) that sometimes gets referred to by other names – such as colon or intestine – but to keep it simple we'll just call it the BOWEL. That's right people, the bowel. I'm hoping that if you say it enough to yourself, you'll remember to send it a Christmas card because it deserves one.

The bowel runs from your stomach – not to be confused with your abdomen – to your anus (a.k.a poo hole) and it's part of your digestive system. It's the escape route for your waste products (you know what I'm talking about). And, to put it in perspective, you need to know what other organs help you digest your food – this is called the 'holistic view'.

Here it is: your digestive system consists of the mouth, teeth, oesophagus, stomach, the small bowel and the large bowel, all the way down to the rectum.

The main job for the bowel is to digest and absorb the water and the nutrients from the food you eat, allowing your body to gather energy and hydrate you for your everyday activities. When your bowel isn't functioning normally, you tend not to absorb your nutrients like you normally would, which means you can start feeling a little tired and sluggish, and you may also notice that you don't tolerate certain foods very well.

Actually, it is not one bowel, but three. The bowel is divided into three different sections and this bit may seem a tad tedious but I'm sure you can apply yourself to the form guide when it suits you, so deal with it. It's important. It's also pretty cool – your human body is so superbly designed that there is nothing else on the planet that matches it.

The small bowel

Its main job is to absorb nutrients from our food once we have digested it. At 2.5 cm in diameter, this part of the bowel is a lot smaller compared with the large bowel, but it's a whopping 5 to 8 metres long, much longer then the larger bowel.

The large bowel (colon)

The colon absorbs water and it has a much wider diameter, 4 to 5 cm, and it's 80 to 100 cm long. It's also prone to cancer.

The rectum

This stores your waste until you are ready to pass it via the anus (i.e. do a poo). It's another area prone to bowel cancer.

On the inside of our small bowel we have little floating string-like things called villi. In a healthy person the villi will remain upright, ready to absorb nutrients from the digested food as it floats past in the small bowel. It's probably not as poetic as it sounds.

When our bowel isn't in good working order, the villi wilt – they lie down instead of standing up – and accordingly they're not able to absorb many of the nutrients from the food. This affects the breakdown of other types of foods, like dairy products, which typically take a bit more work to digest than fruits and vegetables.

I have some clients who have coeliac disease – that is, they can't tolerate wheat or, more specifically, gluten – or who have irritable bowel syndrome, and they're unable to tolerate milk.

If they consume any dairy food they end up feeling bloated or nauseated. It's a definite that their villi aren't working properly, as the tips of the villi hold an important enzyme, called lactase, which helps us to digest and absorb dairy products. Now you've learnt something new for today.

The upkeep

Obviously it's preferable not to experience digestive problems, but often they're the signal that you need to pay a bit more attention to your bowel. It'd be unreal if you could take care of yourself so you never get those signals, but if they've already happened we'll take the better-late-than-never approach.

I'm going to tell you what you need to do to maintain good bowel health and, most importantly, prevent bowel cancer. I like to use this as a worst-case scenario because it usually gets people's attention, but if you prefer you can simply tell yourself that this is what you need to do to prevent the poo from getting so far backed up the shoot that . . . I'm sure you get the idea.

I'm sure these tips will all sound familiar but that's because everyone agrees that they're good. It's time to admit to yourself that absolutely *no one* is going to tell you that eating a pizza while sitting on the couch is good for your parts. Or your poo.

Here are my top tips for healthy poo.

1. Exercise, exercise, exercise. This means walking, running, swimming or playing footy on a regular basis. It does NOT mean walking to the letterbox and back. If you know you don't like solo sweating, join a team. If you get bored doing the same thing every day, then don't. The only rule about exercise is to *do it*.

2. Eat quality lean meats, poultry and fish or plant-based proteins for you non-meat eaters – hamburgers are not in this food group.

3. Eat a variety of vegetables, fruit, whole grain cereals and lentils. This is nowhere near as boring as it sounds – honestly. And you need to eat these foods every day to give you what's known in the trade as *roughage*. See? I didn't mention bran cereal.

4. Eat yoghurts and cheeses.

5. Drink water throughout the day, modifying your intake according to your needs – if you're exercising a lot, you'll need more water than if you're not.

6. Try not to be like everyone else: limit your alcohol intake to one drink per meal. *Do not* save up for a Saturday night blow-out. We all know Aussie blokes like their brew, but there's no beer allowed in hospital. Get the picture?

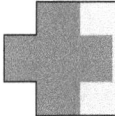

The 50 000 Km service

Here is another *cautionary tale*:

CASE STUDY

My name is Russ Cooper and I have been and still am a Rotarian of some forty years' standing. Around the year 1996 I was asked if I would take on the role of Rotary District Chairman for Rotary Bowelscan. Bowelscan is the selling and testing of pharmaceutical kits for the detection of blood in the stool, which is one of the best ways to diagnose bowel cancer other than by colonoscopy.

I became very involved in this Community Service and held the position until 2006.

I had completed the Bowelscan test in 2005 as was usual, and the results were inconclusive, so I did not worry too much as I had always been clear and my bowel habits had not changed in any major way. This was okay until November that year when I was getting constant bleeding from the rectum every time I had a bowel movement.

I had an appointment with a gastroenterologist to sort out another problem (polyps growing in the gut) so I told him of this problem but added that it was probably from haemorrhoids. The doctor asked if the blood was sticky at all, and I replied that, yes, it was sticky and bright red, which made me think it was haemorrhoids.

He answered that, no, it wasn't haemorrhoids and he would need to do a colonoscopy for a full examination. This was done in January 2006 and the diagnosis was a cancer in the sigmoid area of the colon. He told me that the cancer was up to five years old and was a 'C' on a scale of ABCD – with D the worst – and it did not bleed regularly.

This news shattered my usual peaceful existence. An appointment was made for the next Thursday to see a colorectal surgeon. He informed me that I was in need of major bowel surgery, and quickly. He then added that, as I also suffered from acute angina, I would need to have a cardiologist give me the okay for the operation. The colorectal surgeon phoned my cardiologist then and there and made an appointment for the next Thursday.

The heart specialist listed me in the Lake Macquarie Private Hospital for the next Thursday for an angiogram. This showed that I required four cardiac bypasses before I could undergo the bowel surgery. So I was listed for this operation on the next Thursday in the same hospital. This surgery was successful and I was released to home ten days after the procedure.

Then the wheels fell off. Back to hospital after two days at home to have the left lung drained of 1.75 litres of fluid; as well as the incision on my left leg not healing as well as it should.

To cut a long story short: on the ninth of May 2006 I was admitted to the John Hunter Hospital for major bowel surgery, which was a 'sigmoid colectomy'. Fifteen inches of the bowel were removed which also included a lymph node. When the pathology was completed on the lymph node it proved to be malignant. This then showed that there could be more cancer in my system. So my journey now took in thirty weeks of chemotherapy, every Monday at the Mater Hospital Newcastle.

I must say that I did not suffer too many side effects from this treatment but would have preferred not to have had to have it, but have it I did and now I am seeing my oncologist only once per year and the surgeon only every six months.

My blood counts are excellent and my general heath for a seventy-year-old is okay.

The big thing is that I had a POSITIVE MENTAL ATTITUDE during all of the procedures that I underwent. I was in hospital nine times in 2006, but I am a survivor and I have beaten the Big C. I now live a full life enjoying my only grandchild when I have the chance and am still actively involved in Rotary and Rotary Bowelscan.

Please, if you have any regard for your family, get a Bowelscan kit each year and test yourself for this dreaded disease. Bowel cancer kills more Australians every year than our road toll. It is the biggest cancer-related cause of death in this country and the most easily treated if you can catch it early. So my advice to you men out there is, 'Get off your bum and buy a kit – the life you save will be your own'.

The development of bowel cancer actually takes a number of years. Initially normal little cells within the inside of the bowel become abnormal and multiply, often growing into the form of a polyp (a small lump in the bowel) which over time may develop into a malignant growth – that's another way of saying 'cancer'.

There are three main factors that affect your chances of getting bowel cancer.

1. The older you are, the more likely you are to get it. 'I don't plan to live beyond my thirtieth birthday' is, sadly, not fail-safe.
2. If someone in your family has it, you're at risk. It's as simple as that.
3. Eating badly is like giving cancer a working visa to your bowel.

Polyps will not necessarily become cancerous, but removing them minimises your risk of developing cancer. Because once there are any malignant cells they'll leak small amounts of blood, not detectable by the human eye, before you even see blood in your poo – so you can be fairly far gone by the time you notice. Which is another way of saying (a) prevention really is better than the cure and (b) get yourself checked out regularly if you have any family history or you're over fifty years of age and (c) it's hard to see blood in your poo if you're not actually checking – so just look every now and again. You don't have to be fanatical about it – just be *aware*.

What to look for

Unfortunately, early warning signs of bowel cancer are rare, so these common symptoms listed below are what pop up once the cancer has already developed.

- Bleeding from the rectum. Don't always assume it's just haemorrhoids!
- Altered bowel habits (needing to go to the toilet more or less often/extreme constipation/change in stool shape/ change in consistency).
- Abdominal pain.
- Anaemia (iron deficiency – your gums look white instead of pink, your skin is unusually pale – in other words, you look like a character from *Twilight*.
- Feeling extremely tired.
- Unexplained weight loss (if the cancer has spread).

Who is at risk?

Those most at risk of bowel cancer are people:

- Fifty years or older.
- With a family history of bowel cancer (parent/sibling/child).
- With adenoma polyps in the bowel.
- With Crohn's disease or ulcerative colitis (inflammatory bowel disease).

If you're not in any of those categories, don't completely dismiss your chances of getting it and think you don't have to eat properly or check your poo. There are always exceptions to the rule, and I'm not saying this to scare you – I just want everyone to be as healthy as they can be. It's important to note that, according to the Australian Government Cancer Screening site, up to 75 per cent of people diagnosed with bowel cancer do not have a family history of it.

If you do have a family history, it is EXTREMELY important you have check-ups at an early stage. Often the recommendations for those with a positive family history are to have your first colonoscopy ten years prior to the age your relative was diagnosed, with usually four-to-six yearly follow-ups for the rest of your life.

I once cared for a 52-year-old lady with bowel cancer in Intensive Care. She'd just had 20 cm of her large bowel removed, resulting in the need for a colostomy bag. This lady had two beautiful daughters and a very loving husband, who was retired. I asked her what symptoms she had to make her go to the doctor initially, suspecting something was not quite right. She told me, 'I was bleeding from the backside for two months before I went to the GP. At first it was just specks of blood when I'd wipe my bottom, and I just put it down to a haemorrhoid – not that I'd ever had haemorrhoids before, so I didn't really know what to expect. But as the weeks went by it started to get heavier and the toilet would be filled with red blood – that's when I got worried. I went to the GP and they were really worried. I ended up having a colonoscopy two days later and they found the cancer.'

I asked how she felt about the new addition – the bag – and quite quickly she replied, 'Ah it's nothing. I'm here, aren't I? I get to see my beautiful girls and, I hope, to enjoy retirement with my husband. The bag has meant I can now hopefully have that!'

While I applaud this lady's positive attitude, fellas, I'm fairly confident that you don't want a bag. And the best way to not get a bag is to do exactly as I say and follow those prevention tips and SEE A BLOODY DOCTOR if you're not sure.

Every death from bowel cancer is a tragedy because every cancer was a benign polyp to begin with. If that polyp had been removed, the cancer would not have developed.

If you have symptoms from your bowel, talk to your GP.

If a relative of yours has had bowel cancer, talk to your GP.

If you receive a National Bowel Cancer Screening kit in the mail, don't throw it in the bin.

If you're over 50 – even if you don't have any symptoms, even if none of your relatives has had bowel cancer – talk to your GP about regular FOBTs (Faecal Occult Blood Test).

Dr Cameron Bell
Gastroenterologist
Bowel Cancer and Digestive Research Institute Australia

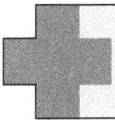

The 150 000 km service

The best possible way to detect bowel cancer is to screen for it. We know bowel cancer can grow slowly for years without showing any signs or symptoms, so it is up to us to find it first.

The whole point to screening for bowel cancer is to find these growths or polyps in their early stages when it is possible to treat, primarily before cancer cells start to form.

One of the best screening tools on the market is a Faecal Occult Blood Test (FOBT). Basically, it is a test you do in your own home, taking two or three consecutive stool specimens and putting them into a container to send to a pathology lab for testing. The test is:

- Cheap.
- User-friendly.
- Confidential.
- Easy to follow.
- Non-invasive.
- Painless.
- Done in your own home.

The test is done to find microscopic traces of blood in the stool, NOT actual bowel cancer. Most cancers and pre-cancers will bleed so the FOBT is an excellent way of identifying these bleeds. According to the Bowel Cancer & Digestive Research Institute Australia, 'If you do a FOBT every two years, you can reduce your risk of dying from bowel cancer by up to one-third.'

The FOBT is not considered 100 per cent accurate due to cancerous cells bleeding microscopic amounts of blood inconsistently, so if you were to give a stool sample one day, it may or may not have blood present, whereas the next sample may have blood present within the stool, therefore you are asked to do two or three samples to minimise the risk of missing a positive test.

Once you do the test at home, you put the samples in a pathology bag and pop it into a designated FOBT collection bin in your community or at your local doctor's surgery.

If the results are positive, your doctor will be notified and you will need to revisit your doctor. But it is important to realise that a positive blood sample does not necessarily mean cancer: it could just mean polyps, inflammation in the bowel, even haemorrhoids. So don't stress – just find out where it's coming from.

The results may actually help you feel *better* about your health. Bet you never thought of that, eh?

I recall one gentleman telling his story of stomach pains ongoing for four to five years. He'd lie in his bed at night occasionally moaning with the discomfort, then suddenly it would go away. His wife once said, 'Love, you've really got to get that seen to'. He replied 'yeah yeah, I'm not a bloody wimp you know, probably nothing more than the food I ate . . .'. Sure enough he told his GP some time later, they did scopes, and found nothing, but the pain was still there and he just kept putting up with it. Finally, he visited another GP some two years later, he mentioned the pains and the ongoing hot flushes he was experiencing. The GP decided to do a few further investigations, when BINGO . . . a CT showed a tumour in his small intestine, and yes, it was malignant, and yes, it had been there for a considerable number of years. Please fellas don't be a wimp, go and get checked out if something *just ain't right*. And if a problem is ongoing, keep asking questions of your doctor.

Getting FOBT

There are a few ways of getting hold of the Faecal Occult Blood Test kits. First, there is the National Bowel Cancer Screening

Program funded by the Australian Government, which is aiming to spread awareness to our community by sending FOBT kits to those turning fifty, fifty-five and sixty-five years of age between January 2008 and December 2010.

I am often asked why every person between the ages of fifty and sixty doesn't have an FOBT kit sent to them automatically. Basically it's because the program is gradually introduced to make sure our medical services can keep up with the potential demand. There is no cost involved to the individual – you simply receive the kit in the mail, take your specimens and send them by mail to the designated pathology lab.

Approximately two weeks after sending the test to the pathology lab the results are sent to you, your nominated doctor and to the National Bowel Cancer Screening Program Register.

For the wider community, there is the Rotary Club Bowelscan kits, which are also FOBT kits. Each year, in conjunction with the National Bowel Cancer Screening Program, Rotary runs the Bowelscan program for one month at a time in your local community, selling these kits for around $8, with a return date for the pathology collection (normally at a designated pharmacy in the area).

Rotary have been on board with this initiative for almost twenty years and, according to Dr Cameron Bell, in 2007 alone 172 cancers and polyps were detected because of this program. Overall 1364 possible cancerous growths and polyps have been detected as a result of the FOBT kits. That's 1364 people whose lives were probably saved because of a simple test. If even one of those people was a friend of yours, that should put it in perspective for you.

You can discuss purchasing an FOBT kit with your doctor or

local pharmacy, or contact Rotary during their program. There are two types of FOBT kits on the market and it's important to follow the instructions specific to each one, as they differ slightly in terms of foods or medications allowed to be taken prior to doing the test.

A positive test means . . .

If your FOBT test gives a positive result – meaning that you have something nasty lurking, you get to have a colonoscopy! I'm using exclamation marks to distract you from the fact that it's not a pleasant procedure!! But it saves lives!!!

The colonoscopy allows a bowel specialist (a gastroenterologist or surgeon) to view the large bowel. The aim is to look for any polyps or abnormal growths on the inside wall of the large bowel by using a long, flexible colonoscope, approximately as wide as your little finger. The word 'colonoscopy' simply refers to the use of a scope to view the colon. Yes! They put a camera up your bum!!! (Still distracted, I hope.) The colonoscope is inserted into the anus, passing through the rectum to the colon in order to have a good gander at the organ.

What you need to do before the camera goes up your date

Before your colonoscopy appointment you'll need to make sure your bowel is completely cleaned out, otherwise the specialist won't be able to see as much of the wall of the bowel as they need. So two days before the procedure you'll be eating and drinking specific foods, avoiding brown bread, high-fibre foods, fruits, vegetables, seeds and nuts, and any yellow cheeses.

The day before the procedure you'll be limited to clear fluids only throughout the day. In the afternoon of the day leading up to the procedure you'll have to drink a preparation drink used for bowel cleansing (your specialist will tell you what it is). Generally you will be asked to drink three lots of the preparation every second hour. This will get your bowels moving – you'll be as clean as a whistle the next day. (Tip: Plan to be home that day!) You won't even know yourself! It's also very important not to eat or drink for six hours prior to the procedure.

Don't worry, you'll get drugs

You'll probably be relieved to learn that you'll be given sedation for the procedure – so much sedation that you'll be sleepy or completely out of it. Before you drop off, though, they'll ask you to lie on your left side for ease of access with the colonoscope. Just remember a colonoscopy is simple and easy compared to what could happen if you ignore the problem.

I'm not going to tell you anything else about the colonoscopy – you'll be asleep, after all. No need for details. All you really need to know is that it takes approximately fifteen to thirty minutes. I'm sure you can imagine what they're doing in that time and if you'd rather not, who can blame you?

The side effects

Colonoscopies are performed in either a hospital or day clinic by a specialist and qualified staff. However, as with all procedures, there's always the possibility of complications. Your doctor can fill you in on these but PLEASE don't let any of these side effects put you off having the colonoscopy, because they aren't commonplace and they're not fatal. Bowel cancer can be fatal.

You need the colonoscopy more than you need to be scared about what could go wrong.

What if they find something?

If the gastroenterologist sees polyps or growths during the procedure, in most cases they will remove the polyps or take a biopsy of the growth, sending it to the pathology lab for analysis. Not all growths or polyps are assumed to be cancerous – they just need to send them to pathology to make sure. And the best part is that you won't feel it if they do remove something. You're sedated, remember?

If the pathology results come through indicating a cancer, usually surgery will be required. If the cancer is in its early stages, there is greater chance of a full recovery. Don't put off having that colonoscopy. I've said this enough times now for you to get the message.

What if there's nothing there?

If the results are all clear and there are no growths or polyps, then this means you have a low risk of developing bowel cancer over the next ten years. But since you're only having the colonoscopy because you had a positive FOBT result, you should still do regular FOBTs and if you do have any sneaking suspicion or symptoms of bowel cancer, see your doctor immediately. Not seeing the doctor does *not* make your symptoms go away.

But wait . . . there's more!

Your doc may suggest that you also have a gastroscopy, which is a procedure to check the small bowel.

As the name suggests, the gastroscopy involves a camera going down your mouth into your gastrointestinal system – into your oesophagus and stomach, then down into the small bowel.

The gastroscopy looks for signs of polyps, ulcers and tumours or areas of bleeding in the stomach, oesophagus and the small bowel.

The preparations are a bit easier than those for a colonoscopy – all you need to do is not eat for six hours prior to the procedure.

More drugs!

You get to be asleep for a gastroscopy too – no one really wants to feel a scope going into their mouth. This test takes approximately ten minutes, so you'll have a nice short nap and wake up none the wiser.

The not-so-good night's sleep

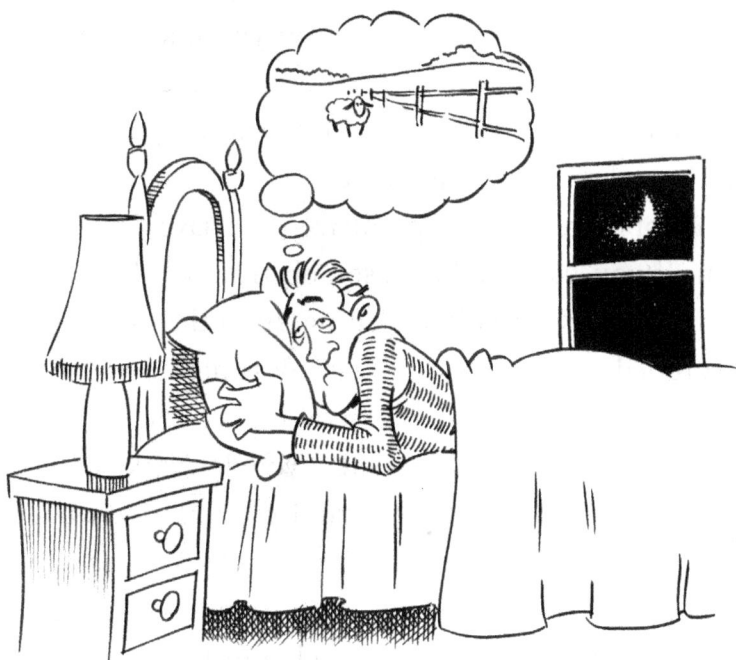

We all have a bad night's sleep every now and again. But if you're waking up every morning – *every single morning* – feeling tired and cranky, plus you're generally just low in energy, there's a good chance you're sleeping really badly. And I'm not talking about snoring.

Blokes get a bad rap for snoring, but they're no more likely to snore than women. It's just that you lot are more likely to have sleep apnoea – a 'super-snoring' condition that can be life threatening. Sleep apnoea doesn't have to be a permanent condition, though – you can take a few simple steps to prevent it or get rid of it, and you'll not only get much better sleep (which will improve the quality of your life overall) but you'll get back in the good books of the poor person sharing your bed.

If you have a partner, she (or he – I don't know what your preferences are!) may find your sleep apnoea extremely frightening, as she/he lies listening to you taking one large, roaring breath after another . . . then nothing. Five or ten seconds can pass and all of a sudden you'll be struggling for your next breath. On and on it goes, all night.

You not only have a sleep problem – you have a relationship problem. If you have undiagnosed obstructive sleep apnoea, your partner will be regularly getting up in the morning tired and frustrated after yet another sleepless night, while you're none the wiser. It's a chain of bloody misery and it's going to affect every single thing in your life if you don't take care of it.

Think about it. If you're tired and your partner's tired all the time then you're both going to be cranky with each other, with the kids, if you have them, with friends and colleagues. This will start to impact on your relationships, making you more miserable than you already are. Apart from that, sleep deprivation has a damaging effect on your body. Every single person on this planet needs a certain amount of sleep for the body to repair itself, grow new cells and digest food. If you're not getting the sleep, your body systems will start to play up. So you're tired, sick and cranky every single day. Nobody wants to live like that. Why are you still doing it?

You could think of sleep apnoea as being like a hole in your car exhaust. At first you don't really know it exists as you can only hear it some of the time. But gradually the noise gets worse, and people soon start to complain, yet you're still getting from A to B, so why bother fixing it? Well, the reason is that your car's not running properly and eventually it'll just stop.

What is obstructive sleep apnoea?

When we sleep our entire body relaxes. If you have obstructive sleep apnoea, not only does the body relax, so does the soft tissue in the back of your throat, causing it to block the windpipe close to your tongue, limiting the amount of air going into your lungs.

'Apnoea' simply means to stop breathing for anywhere from a few seconds to up to a minute.

With limited air getting into your lungs while you are asleep, you unconsciously start taking shallower breaths, which often results in snoring. Taking shallower breaths or no breaths at all for frequent periods throughout the night causes your oxygen levels within the blood to fall. This is the main problem.

Often the question I'm asked is, 'So, what are you saying? I just stop breathing and won't wake up again – next minute I'm dead?' Well, not exactly, because your body is smarter than you think it is. Your brain senses that you're not breathing due to the low levels of oxygen in your blood. It will wake you briefly, and instantly the soft tissue lifts from the back of the throat, allowing air to flow into the windpipe again. But you can imagine that if you are obstructing the airflow many times throughout the night, you will not be getting much quality sleep.

How to tell if you have sleep apnoea

This simple list can help you identify if you're spending your nights wrestling with the sleep demon. You may have:

- poor concentration.
- feel irritable.
- fatigue, feel constantly tired.
- changes in moods.
- high blood pressure.
- impotence.
- low libido (sex drive).

If those last two items aren't enough to get your attention, I'm out of tricks. Yes, gents, when you're tired your little fella gets tired too and he won't come out and play so happily. Your little fella, or should I just say 'fella', needs a good blood supply – a good *oxygenated* blood supply.

Sleep apnoea is NOT another word for snoring

The reason most people go for a check-up and are initially diagnosed with obstructive sleep apnoea is because partners complain about the noise during the night, assuming it is snoring.

Snoring is a different issue and there are certainly steps you can take to minimise the problem, such as:

- losing weight (yes, you);
- limiting alcohol intake before going to bed (no nightcaps);
- clearing the nasal passages.

When I first started working as a nurse in Sydney I used to do a second job on Friday nights in a private plastic surgery clinic, where we would see many women and very few men. The main reason for the male admissions was for a rhinoplasty – basically, a nose job.

Usually the patient had a nasal passage that had become blocked, causing them to snore, and therefore they had the surgery to fix the problem. Often these guys would tell me that they only started snoring after they had their nose broken in a footy game, or other minor incidents, so they didn't want to get surgery until they had stopped playing altogether. And while this may be your situation too, a nose job will not stop the snoring if you carry too much body weight!

Why is sleep apnoea such a concern?

Quite apart from annoying your partner to the extreme, let's further explore sleep apnoea's main detrimental effects.

1. Reducing the amount of oxygen in your bloodstream – last time I checked we need oxygen to stay alive. A drop in your oxygen saturation levels over a prolonged period can put you at risk of high blood pressure, heart attack and stroke. I'm fairly sure you're not putting your hand up for those little party poopers.

2. Increased work of the lungs and brain in breathing – if you overuse your parts, they wear out. Moreover, whenever a body part works it uses energy – if your lungs are working overnight at a rate they're not designed to maintain, your energy levels will drop.

3. Poor quality sleep – this means you don't get your REM (rapid eye movement) sleep, which is crucial for human health, and you become tired all the time. Fatigue caused by ongoing poor sleep can take the form of:

- Feeling foggy in the brain.
- Feeling exhausted before you even start your day.
- Feeling tired all the time.
- Lethargy.
- 'Can't be bothered' attitude.
- Micro-sleeps while driving, which increase the risk of an accident.

Here's something you probably haven't considered. If you're suffering from even one of these symptoms, you present an occupational health and safety risk. Undiagnosed obstructive sleep apnoea has been linked with incidents in the workplace (purely due to the lack of concentration), and a higher rate of motor vehicle accidents.

I often hear men in their workplace laughing at one of their colleagues, calling them names that suggest the colleague is 'lazy' and 'unmotivated', with a bit of extra language for colour – no doubt you know what I mean . . . But what if the bloke has sleep apnoea? Of course, he could be bone lazy, but sleep apnoea won't help the situation. And no one wants to be thought of as a shirker.

How bad can sleep apnoea get?

Sleep apnoea can be diagnosed as mild, moderate to severe.
- Mild sleep apnoea – five to fifteen disturbed breathing periods an hour.
- Moderate sleep apnoea – fifteen to thirty disturbed breathing periods an hour.
- Severe sleep apnoea – over thirty disturbed breathing periods an hour.

Allow me to tell you a little story about one gentleman.

CASE STUDY

This gent was sixty-six years of age and was recently told that he needed to undergo a sleep study in order to see whether he may have sleep apnoea.

He weighed 135 kg, experienced a heart attack back in 2002, had ongoing chest discomfort (angina) for four years before that, and suffered from extremely high blood pressure of around 190/112mmHg on average (which is pretty bloody high) and continued to be highly medicated for this condition.

This gentleman travelled throughout New South Wales, driving heavy vehicles, covering up to 2000 km per week, and frequently needed to have other people travel with him because of his fatigue. 'I just can't keep my eyes open,' he told me, 'I don't know what it is. I normally go through a bag of Minties to keep me awake in a three-hour trip.'

The reason that his doctor had requested a sleep study was because of a day clinic procedure during which an anaesthetist had needed to look at this gentleman's oxygen level.

If you have ever been in hospital you'll know that a little device called the oximetry or saturation probe is placed on a finger in order to get a reading of how much oxygen is circulating the body in the blood. In healthy individuals the level is 96 to 100 per cent saturation, while smokers or people with lung disease such as emphysema may have saturations of 88 to 92 per cent. This particular patient had saturations of 78 per cent while lying on his back, wide awake, having a chat. The doctor was concerned as this man had purple-looking lips and bluish/purple legs, basically a sign that he had very little oxygen getting around his body and, more importantly, his head and his heart.

The man agreed that he was a snorer, and complained of being tired all the time and generally feeling unwell; he felt that his body 'just wasn't coping'.

He agreed to having the sleep study, which would involve staying overnight in a sleep clinic, where a technician could oversee what happened to both the brainwaves and the amount of oxygen the patient would get while sleeping the way they normally would.

Severe sleep apnoea is diagnosed if the person stops breathing thirty times in one hour. This gentleman managed to have seventy-five apnoeic episodes per hour. Therefore, on average he woke more than once per minute due to not breathing, and his average oxygen saturation was 63 per cent throughout his sleep.

His heart was working overtime in order to get enough blood with enough oxygen to service all of his body. Something had to give – and you could literally see it on the patient's body.

This man needed positive pressure to his airway while asleep, to stop his airway from obstructing (closing in) and allow oxygen to enter his body. This 'positive pressure' refers to a machine called CPAP, otherwise known as Continuous Positive Airway Pressure.

I'm hoping you haven't already turned purple – and if you have I'd suggest you put down this book immediately and run to your nearest doctor. But it's more likely that you've realised that it's preferable to prevent the apneoa *before* you get to the purple stage. If you think you're having problems with sleep – or your partner tells you that you do – don't ignore it hoping it will all end some day. Living with extreme tiredness and low oxygen levels is just going to make everything miserable. You wouldn't put sugar in your petrol tank, would you? Yeah, I thought not. Sleep apnoea is the sugar in your tank.

Pull up your socks

You are at risk of obstructive sleep apnoea if you are:

- **Obese** – carrying extra weight increases the likelihood of snoring and apnoeic episodes while you sleep. Obesity often causes people to appear to have a short, thick neck due to the fatty tissue lining the region, which also causes narrowing of the throat. Just imagine what happens when that fatty tissue lies down to sleep at night – can't you just see it squashing the windpipe? Stop wondering whether you need to lose weight; the wondering days are over. If you have sleep apnoea, are overweight and lose 10 to 15 kilograms, you can dramatically improve the quality of your sleep.
- **Male** – men are three times more likely to have sleep apnoea then women. Don't bother whinging about it – accept it and realise that you are at greater risk.
- **An alcohol and sedative user** – these are both muscle relaxants which will increase your risk of apnoea and snoring. Yes, it's fun to drink beer. Just do it in moderation for a change.
- **A smoker** – smoking causes inflammation to your throat and your airway.

You are also at risk if you have:

- **Abnormal hormone levels** affecting the thyroid, causing diabetes, or indicating excessive amounts of growth hormone.

- **Blocked nose** – snoring and apnoea at times are often caused by a broken nose/trauma to the nose, hayfever or inflamed sinuses.
- **Cranio-facial abnormalities** – jaws that are not in alignment can obstruct the airway and cause further damage to your teeth. Often surgery is the preferred option.

If you think all this sounds familiar . . .

Visit your GP and explain what symptoms you've been having or what your partner has been witnessing. The GP should refer you to a lung doctor (respiratory specialist) who may wish to do lung function tests and possibly send you for a sleep study in a sleep disorders clinic.

This is not such a bad gig – you just turn up and go to sleep. It's the researchers who do all the work. Generally you arrive at the sleep clinic on your appointed day in time to eat an evening meal and continue with what you would normally do if you were at home. You're usually advised to bring your own pillow, or if you normally drink a beer or wine with or after your meal to notify staff in order for them to organise this (this is the case in most sleep clinics anyway). The aim is to make this as similar to your everyday routine as possible.

For the next step, the sleep technicians will attach electrodes to your chest and head to monitor your heart rhythm and to assess how often you breathe throughout the night. A pulse oximetry (probe to measure your oxygen saturation) is applied to your finger or ear allowing the technicians to see the amount of oxygen in your blood throughout your sleep. Your job is to sleep. At 7 a.m. you can go home – although it's possible you may not want to, since they supply all that food and wine . . .

Your specialist will tell you the results of the sleep study, determining whether you have sleep apnoea and whether or not you need further treatment.

If you do need further treatment, such as wearing a CPAP mask (see p71), you will have to come into the sleep disorder clinic again to trial the mask and learn how to use it. This also allows the technician to adjust the mask and determine how much pressure you need to keep your airway open.

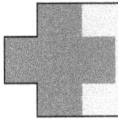

The 50 000 Km service

I've already mentioned some things you can do to treat sleep apnoea, but it's probably worth running through them again to make sure you're really, truly getting it. It is crucial to take care of this condition if you have it – we probably don't even know the full extent of sleep apnoea on the health and wellbeing of sufferers and their families.

There are a number of steps you can take to treat sleep apnoea, from lifestyle changes to surgery, medications and wearing a mask. The treatment depends on the status of your health.

We'll go through what you'll probably consider to be the 'boring bit' first. If you've read other chapters then the information will look very familiar. That's because the recommendations for maintaining good health are universally accepted: eat well and exercise. EAT WELL AND EXERCISE. How many times do I have to tell you? Okay, just once more.

The first step to take when treating sleep apnoea.

1. Make changes to your everyday habits.

- lose excess body fat

- limit alcohol intake – note that I said 'limit' not 'stop'
- stop smoking
- stop taking sedatives – make sure you do this in consultation with your doctor
- start exercising – happily, playing footy counts as exercise.

Some other steps to take, which may or may not apply to you.

2. Have surgery to correct cranio-facial abnormalities/obstructions.

3. Correct abnormal hormone levels.

4. Wear a mouthguard.

5. Wear a CPAP mask while sleeping.

The spare parts

Mouth splint

A mouthguard or mouth splint props the jaw forward, helping to reduce the effects of both sleep apnoea and snoring. For many people this works well, as long as they also have strong, healthy teeth for the correct positioning of the plate.

CPAP (Continuous Positive Airway Pressure)

This is a pump that delivers a set pressure of air through a long hoselike tube to a mask which is positioned either over your nose or your face. You wear it while you sleep, whenever you sleep – night/ day/ naps, etc. The machine forces a positive pressure through your nose or mouth into the back of your throat, ensuring it remains open, allowing air to reach your lungs while you are sleeping. Generally CPAP is used for those with

moderate to severe sleep apnoea, and it's a fantastic invention which has saved and prolonged many people's lives.
Sourced – Adelaide Institute for Sleep Health – Using your CPAP at home, 2007.

Once your CPAP mask is fitted to your face properly and you are able to tolerate the pressure required to keep your airway open while you sleep, you will notice improvements to both your energy level and your sleep.

What you need to know when using a CPAP mask?

Even though this might sound like commonsense, it is really important not to eat or drink while using the CPAP mask. If you wear a face mask, it is recommended by sleep clinics not to eat a large meal two to three hours before going to sleep.

When you are diagnosed with sleep apnoea, you need to start viewing the CPAP mask as part of your daily routine, like brushing your teeth. If you are travelling, or intending to sleep elsewhere other than home (not making any judgements here, tiger!), take it with you. The machine is small enough to be packed into a bag. And if you're worrying about the noise, don't. These days most machines are super quiet.

But don't take it from me . . .

CASE STUDY

I commenced using CPAP in 2001 after a clinic confirmed sleep apnoea, with me stopping breathing many times each hour while I was asleep. I was having difficulty using CPAP during 2002, as evidenced by being unable to control blood pressure during that period.

After having the machine adjusted by the supplier it has been easier to use and much more effective, resulting in my blood pressure being well controlled in recent years.

Since 2002 I have experienced no difficulty in using the machine and it is second nature to put the mask on every time before settling down for a good and restful sleep each night. My energy levels have increased significantly over the period of CPAP usage.

It has been suggested that the machine would be a 'romance killer' but I don't necessarily agree with that.

Barry Daniels, Retiree (clearly an *active* retiree)

Is CPAP comfortable to use?

There are a few concerns for people when it comes to using a CPAP machine, such as the fitting of the mask, the positive pressure felt when breathing in and out of the nose and mouth, dryness of the throat and the sensation.

When using the CPAP, some people have commented that the pressure feels too high in order to breathe out, giving them the sensation that they are unable to breathe. It may feel very foreign to you, but if you persist you'll get used to the sensation, it can take some people one to two weeks, others a little longer.

The CPAP mask is comfortable or tolerable once the mask has been correctly fitted to your face and the pressure adjusted according to what you need.

Don't get me wrong, CPAP can be very uncomfortable if the mask is not fitting your face securely, and this is why you can choose between a face mask and a nasal mask. Often this is a reason fellas don't bother wearing CPAP at all due to the discomfort factor, but it is a matter of persisting and trialling lots of varieties until you are comfortable. And it's worth it.

If this is all sounding like too much hard work, review the symptoms and effects of sleep apnoea listed on p62 and then tell me whether you want to continue to live like that. Then review the other things you can do to improve your health and realise that if you do those things, you may not need the CPAP.

How long will I have to use it?

This will be up to your doctor. Often when people change their lifestyle by either losing weight or starting to exercise, their sleep apnoea can improve to a point where the CPAP pressures can be decreased or not used at all. But many people will need to use this machine for the rest of their life. If this turns out to be you, try to see the positive side of it – an invention that can save your life. It's not something anyone, apart from your nearest and dearest, need to see – pets can be very forgiving.

What changes will I see by using it?

CPAP will help you:

- Achieve the ability to sleep.
- Reduce high blood pressure levels.
- Improve ongoing disturbed sleep.
- Feel energised after sleeping.
- Prevent snoring (hurrah!).

The bottom line is that there is treatment for sleep apnoea, between CPAP and some lifestyle tweaks, you can be living a much improved life, with plenty of oomph for all the fun stuff

– and if that isn't a good enough reason to take care of yourself, well . . .

The big yawn

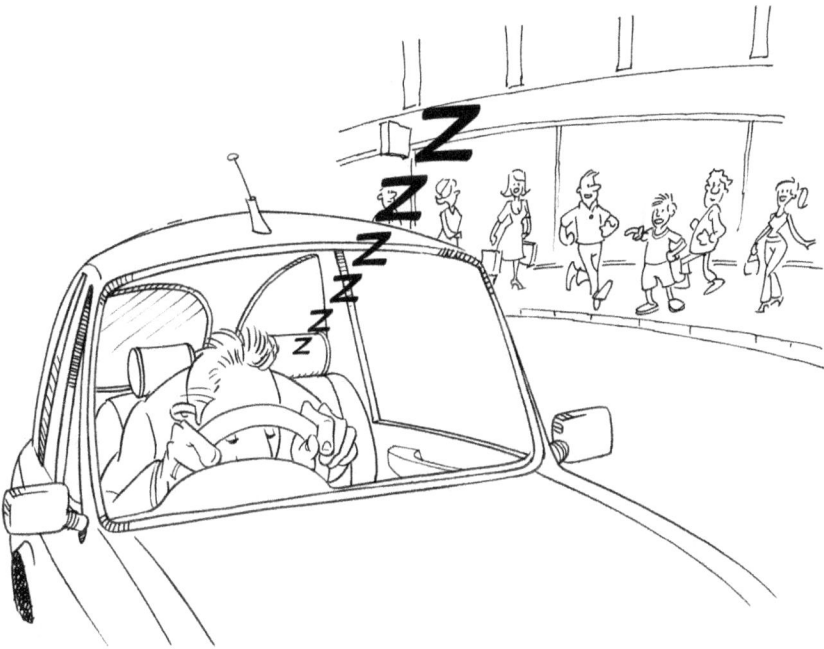

We all get tired. Whether we've been studying all night or partying till dawn, or just doing too much and not getting enough rest. We've all had days when yawning is our main form of exercise. Sometimes tiredness becomes a habit – we have made some incremental changes in our lifestyle and suddenly we're sleeping less than we need and probably having poor-quality sleep when we finally do hit the sack. This is when you start to suffer from fatigue. And fatigue can kill you.

The causes

Fatigue – in a medical sense – can be a result of workplace expectations, personal commitments, health problems, an active social life without balance and changes to family life.

More specifically, fatigue can develop as a result of:
- Poor workplace rostering.
- Ongoing stress.
- Working extra jobs.
- Jetlag.
- Lack of sleep.
- Emotional/family issues.
- Unhealthy habits.
- Shift work – our body clock uses sunshine as a prompt to be active and alert, so if this response becomes confused we often cannot get to sleep.
- Not eating adequate amounts of food.
- Drugs and alcohol.
- Medical concerns, such as glandular fever, anaemia, coeliac disease, sleep disorders, chronic fatigue syndrome, chronic pain, myalgic encephalopathy, hypothyroidism, cancer, heart problems, hepatitis, Parkinson's disease and HIV.
- Depression, anxiety, grief.
- Unsettled sleep.
- Feeling burnt out.
- Inactivity.
- A snoring companion.

• Getting too much sleep (over 11 hours per day).

No doubt you've just read that list and been able to tick several items – I sure have. If you think about it, though, it's likely those things that apply to you didn't all happen at once. If they did, you'd probably be fatigued because there's only so much a human body can withstand. But if it's one thing – or even two – at a time, you can probably cope. At any rate, let's look a bit more closely at how you'll know you're fatigued.

The signs

Symptoms of fatigue differ for each person. Generally the warning signs include:
• Slowed reflexes and responses.
• Dizziness.
• Blurry vision.
• Poor attention span.
• Headache.
• Moodiness.
• Sore or aching muscles.
• Impaired decision-making and judgement.
• Appetite loss.
• Chronic tiredness or sleepiness.
• Short-term memory problems.
• Poor concentration.
• Low motivation.
• Poor hand-to-eye coordination.

The effects

You may not love your job, but it will be the first thing to suffer if you're fatigued. And your job provides money, so it's probably not a good idea to muck around with it. Fatigue can be especially dangerous if you are a tradie or working in a job that involves a lot of manual labour. So remember the following effects of fatigue are serious.

- Loss of concentration.
- Vehicle or heavy machinery accidents.
- Workplace accidents.
- Critical mistakes in the workplace.
- Poor judgement.
- Insomnia.

There are also some facts you need to think about.

- Every day, driver drowsiness kills at least one person on Australian roads.
- Road accidents cost Australians an estimated $15 billion a year.
- 28 per cent of heavy vehicle licence holders reported having fallen asleep while driving.
- Drivers with less than six hours of sleep are 2.5 times more likely to doze off.
- In 2007, one in five drivers reported experiencing events such as dozing off, near misses and crossing lanes.
- Up to 30 per cent of truck fatalities and 52 per cent of major crash insurance claims are fatigue related.
- Working 50 hours or more per week has become more common for full-time workers over the last 20 years, at a

rate of 30 per cent up from 22 per cent in 1985.
*Source: National Transport Commission research published by
Vic Roads* http://studio.optalert.com/www.abs.gov.au

What, me tired?

Fatigue can affect us all. While you're reading about fatigue, bear in mind it applies to the other people around you, driving their cars or their trucks because of a tight deadline, or the colleagues handling massive equipment while you work alongside them, or the hospital staff who are attempting to save your life or the life of someone you love – even the bus driver or pilot ferrying people to their destination. What if your bus driver or doctor hadn't slept for twenty hours – do you think they're going to be working safely?

How often do people push themselves too hard and decide to start an eight-hour drive after a day at work, especially at those times of the year when you're aiming to get away on holidays, or on a Friday night and you only have the weekend away to play? We've all done it. You've done it, haven't you? And you've probably bragged about it – 'I made Melbourne in seven hours with only one wee break'. Yeah, you're a champion. You're also an idiot, because it's only by the grace of some all-knowing and wise Being without a Name that you're still with us. That kind of driving bravado kills people. 'Stop, revive, survive' is a good slogan not just because it's catchy – it's also *true*.

Every time I get into a taxi I always start my general chat with the driver by saying, 'So how long have you been working for today?' I'm genuinely interested in the answer, but I'm also trying to gauge the level of safety in the car. If the cabbie tells you, 'I am on to my fifteenth hour', start saying your Hail Marys, unless you feel like getting out of the car right away. In 2009, there was an article in the *Sydney Morning Herald* (Paul Bibby, 4 January 2009) which looked at taxi drivers working 24-hour shifts over the holiday season to pull in some extra cash; they could make anywhere up to $1000 a day if they could work a full twenty-four hours with only a sixty-minute break. The NSW Transport Minister, David Campbell, described this as 'dangerous and plain stupid', with some drivers pushing through fatigue at a time when the city's roads are at their most crowded, breaching all regulations.

Imagine being in the car with one of those dudes. Imagine *being* one of those dudes. As the president of the Australasian College of Road Safety, Lauchlan McIntosh, stated in the *Herald* article, 'It's not only the drivers who are at risk from this behaviour but also the customer and other road users.'

But it isn't just cabbies who clock up long hours. Don't underestimate the impact on businessmen who are expected to travel for a day to attend one meeting and then fly back that very same day. So not only are they flying – with all the wear and tear on the body that that entails – but they're expected to walk in the office door at either end of the trip. There is a physical and mental cost to pushing your body too hard.

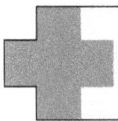

The 50 000 Km service

Now that I've scared the bejesus out of you, let's have a look at the mechanics of fatigue.

Your body clock is otherwise known as your circadian rhythm.

'Circadian' refers to a one-day cycle – your circadian rhythm is programmed to work over a set 24-hour period. When your body detects sunlight, messages are sent to the brain's neuro-transmitters and the body produces chemicals such as melatonin, which prompt your body to coordinate its daily functions. If you ever need to go to the toilet as soon as you wake up, that's why. The circadian rhythm affects your sleep, body temperature, energy levels, libido, the amount of hormones released, your blood pressure, heart rate, mood and digestion.

If you are suffering from fatigue, your circadian rhythm will be affected, and so too will all of these bodily functions. And you can imagine how much fun you won't be having if sleep and digestion alone are not working probably – not only are you getting two hours' shut-eye a night, but you can't poo!

The best way to avoid this kind of disruption is to prevent fatigue becoming chronic in the first place. And to do this you need to identify the reason for the fatigue.

Many blokes might complain they are tired – 'I'm not sleeping because I've been doing night duty for five nights in a row and I only ever average three hours of sleep during the day'. Lack of sleep is an obvious – and very common – reason why a person becomes fatigued over time. If it goes on long enough it becomes sleep debt and you can never repay sleep debt no matter how hard you try, or how many more hours you sleep to make up for it. As facile as it sounds, the best thing to do is to *not lose sleep*. In fact, it's critical for your health. Don't think you're tough if you're only sleeping three hours a night. You're not – you're just damaging yourself and making life dangerous for people around you, particularly if you work in an industry that uses heavy machinery.

Maybe you think you're getting enough sleep, and you're still exhausted. It may be that you have poor sleep quality – you dream a lot, or you're restless, or you have **Sleep Apnoea** (there's a chapter on that in this book – how useful!). You may dream a lot because of something else going on in your life such as being stressed.

Another reason for fatigue is that you're overworking your body and not giving it enough of a chance to rest. If you have a really physical job – you're hauling bricks all day – or you exercise a lot (say, you run 20 kilometres each day) then your body needs the proper nutrition and adequate rest. If you don't get that then, over time, your body will fatigue.

If you're really having trouble working out why you're fatigued – although I reckon most people can work it out if they take five minutes to look at their lifestyle – then ask your missus or your mother (they'd probably have a fair idea), or go to your doctor or, if you prefer, a naturopath and chat to them about it.

Once you know the reason for your fatigue, you can take steps to improve the situation. You may need to change your surroundings – if you're a shift worker sleeping during the day, try to make the room as dark as possible, but with as much circulation or breeze in order to minimise overheating and waking as a result. If you're waking due to noise – your teenage son plays the drums till 2 a.m. or you're in a noisy apartment building – use earplugs. Quite often there's a simple solution – you just need to investigate and find it.

The checklist

Here's my fairly simple list for fighting fatigue.

1. Question the cause of why you are unable to sleep.
2. Take steps to help the situation.
3. If there is a medical condition, seek medical advice in alleviating this problem.
4. Eat nutritious foods daily and don't grumble about it.
5. Ensure you are hydrated throughout the day before going to sleep – beer does not count as hydration. Only water counts.
6. Keep physically active, that means doing some exercise.
7. Limit your alcohol intake, caffeine and cigarettes, especially before going to sleep. A nightcap can be counterproductive.

Some extra tips to help ease fatigue

- Use your bedroom for sleeping and sexual activities only. Get rid of the TV and don't use the bed as a place to spread out the household accounts. Your body and mind needs to view this room as a place of relaxation and peace.
- Listen to your body and go to sleep when you're tired (don't try to get through the last twenty minutes of your favourite TV show – that's what DVDs are for).
- Try not to have afternoon naps if this is preventing you from sleeping at night.
- Attempt to develop a routine with your sleeping pattern, such as waking at the same time every day (although this can obviously be difficult when working in rotating shift work).
- Get adequate sunlight throughout the day, as this helps to regulate your body clock. Five minutes here or there will do it.
- Ensure that you're comfortable when you sleep. This may mean that you need a better bed, a quieter partner (ha ha)

or even a set of earplugs, or thicker curtains to keep the room darkened.

- If you have a family or friendly neighbours, make sure they all know you are on shift work, the phones can be turned down or off, and post a sign on your bedroom door.
- Don't eat for at least an hour or so before going to sleep, if you eat a heavy meal it can keep you awake.
- If you have a 'busy head', do some relaxation exercises to help your mind switch off at the end of the day. This can include reading a novel that takes your mind to another place or practising breathing exercises. There are lots of relaxation CDs around. Please note that Metallica CDs are not in this category.
- Take a look at your diet. Ask yourself whether the foods you eat give you the get up and go you require. You need to:

> **a.** eat breakfast – lots of people skip breakfast but it's a bad bad bad thing to do;
>
> **b.** eat nutritious food – I've said it before and I'll say it again, there's just no substitute for fruit and veg;
>
> **c.** eat meals regularly throughout the day;
>
> **d.** eat sufficient iron-based foods, to prevent anaemia – you'll be pleased to know that eating steak counts;
>
> **e.** drink plain water, not flavoured water;
>
> **f.** drink no more than two caffeinated drinks per day;
>
> **g.** avoid 'dieting' by eating low-kilojoule foods, which give you little energy to keep in reserve;
>
> **h.** keep foods with high fat, high salt and high sugar to a minimum (as these foods do not have the energising effect on the body);

i. drink a warm glass of milk at night before going to sleep – it can help you become 'sleepy'.

The occupational health and safety types are turning somersaults trying to help workers prevent fatigue. There's all sorts of technology coming onto the market – one company allows their workers to wear a watch that monitors their heart rate, sensing periods when the body's functions are slowing down and sends warning signals of fatigue. Another company uses glasses which appear to be safety glasses but can actually sense how often the employee is blinking. This type of technology alerts a driver to potential drowsiness, giving them the opportunity to take a rest rather than pushing through to the next hour, possibly putting themselves and others at risk.

Here are some facts to help you understand why this OHS stuff is important:

- Ninety-three per cent of haulage truck accidents are a result of human error;
- Seventy per cent of human error accidents are related to drowsiness or fatigue.

Optalert Promotional Information sheets <u>*www.optalert.com*</u>

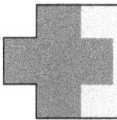

The 150 000 km service

You may have heard of chronic fatigue. Although it is not all that common, you certainly know when a person is suffering from it.

Chronic fatigue is also known as myalgic encephalomyelitis, an illness causing exhaustion, pain to the muscles and possible inflammation in the brain and spinal cord, affecting both adults and children.

Chronic fatigue can occur suddenly or after trauma or viral infections (such as glandular fever), in which case it can develop slowly. Exposure to toxic substances can also place a person at risk of chronic fatigue over time. Fundamentally, though, there is no single known cause.

The effects of chronic fatigue can vary for each person, with one experiencing fatigue-like symptoms and muscle aches, whereas others can barely walk from the bedroom to the bathroom without feeling the need to rest.

The common symptoms include:

- Exhaustion.
- Persistent lack of energy.
- Poor memory and thinking ability.
- Pain.
- Poor sleep.
- Shortness of breath while exercising or otherwise pushing yourself.
- Lowered blood pressure when standing.
- Fast heart rate when standing.
- Palpitations.
- Muscle twitching and tingling.
- Allergies and food intolerances.
- Sore throat, sensitive lymph nodes.
- Fluctuation in weight.
- Sensitive to changes in temperature.
- Nausea and tummy upsets.
- Urinary problems.

These symptoms will vary throughout the illness. And if you have any of them you need to take them seriously: don't try to push yourself at every opportunity as you can experience relapses, and the fatigue may actually worsen.

The difficulty of having an illness like chronic fatigue is that it can be hard to officially diagnose and the sufferer tends to feel frustrated at not being able to carry out normal everyday activities they used to do.

The illness can stop people from attending work, school, special occasions, nights out and just general living. If you're suffering from this type of exhaustion it seems likely that you might have chronic fatigue. It is really important to see your doctor for advice on what to do, even if you get some much needed support. A nutritionist can also help you make the best food choices to help your body heal.

Jetsetter's fatigue

Jet lag is caused by your body travelling across different time zones and fatigue from the trip.

As we already know, the circadian rhythm keeps your bodily functions set to a 24-hour cycle, so when this cycle is disturbed you can feel very tired and completely out of sorts. If you've ever flown across more than a couple of time zones, you'll know what I mean (going to Bali doesn't really do it).

The common signs of jet lag are:

- Fatigue.
- Insomnia.
- Feeling low.
- Poor appetite and nausea.

- Headache.
- Dehydration.
- Poor digestion.
- Tiredness.
- Forgetfulness.
- Poor judgement.
- Poor decision making.
- Irritability.

Kind of makes you want to not travel, dunnit? But the benefits tend to outweigh the bad stuff. Unless you've been in India and had Delhi Belly *during* your trip.

Tips to reduce the effects of jet lag

The biggest and best tip would be to only travel within a couple of time zones, which means going no further than New Zealand or Singapore. Or Perth, if you're on the Australian east coast. So now we've discounted that . . .

Remember that jet lag can affect each of us in different ways. According to the team at Better Health Channel and the Department of Psychology at Waikato Hospital, New Zealand, each of us will experience and recover from jet lag at different times. Here are a few recommended handy hints.

1. If possible, sleep before you get on the plane. Do not 'save it all up' for the plane, because you may not – in fact, you probably won't – sleep.
2. Make sure you wear clothes that are comfortable and non-restrictive.
3. Walk along the aisle whenever possible and perform calf stretches to help your circulation and prevent the risk of

deep vein thrombosis.

4. Nap on the plane whenever you feel the need.
5. Wear eye masks or earplugs to block out light and noise.
6. Try to arrive at your destination at night to help your body adjust to the new time zone.
7. Make sure to keep up your water intake to minimise dehydration and the headaches which can be a part of jet lag.
8. Keep alcohol to a minimum during your flight; you might drift off to sleep but you will wake feeling unrested and dehydrated.
9. Once you have arrived at your destination – and, hopefully, had a kip – expose yourself to sunlight, this will help you stay wide awake.
10. If you decide to use sleeping tablets, make sure you talk to your doctor about this before you fly.

Everyone has their own personal jet lag tricks but I suspect that we all suffer from it, regardless of what we try to do. It's the penalty we pay for living on the other side of the world and a whole hemisphere away from most travel destinations. But it's kind of nice down here, so it's worth it.

What every bloke needs to know about mental un-health

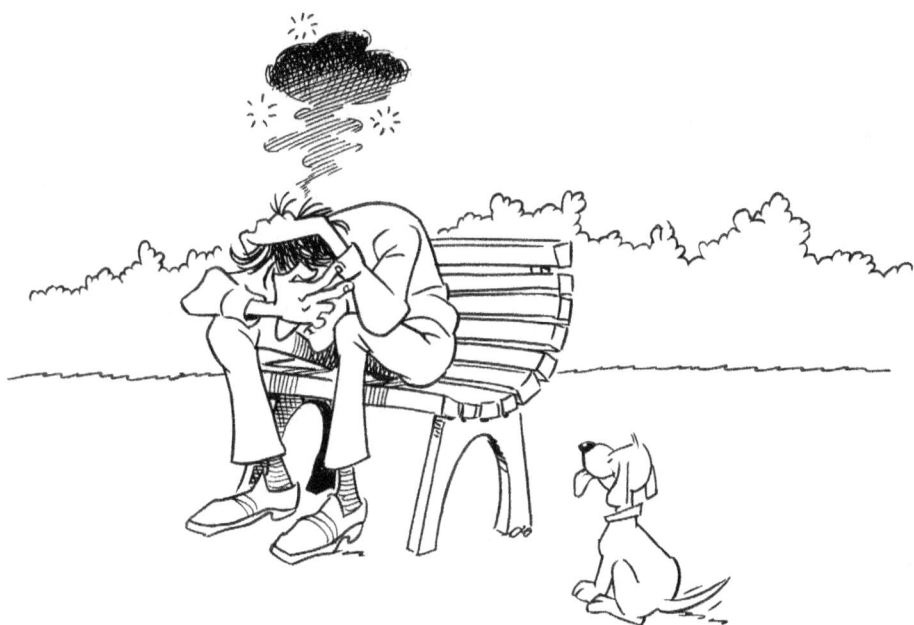

The term 'mental health' can be a problem because we're really talking about mental un-health, aren't we? We're talking about:

- Depression.
- Anxiety.
- Bipolar disorder.

- Stress.
- Anger.
- Insomnia.
- Suicidal thoughts.
- Alcohol abuse.
- Physical abuse.
- Grief.

Can you honestly say that NONE of these has ever happened to you? I wouldn't mind betting you can tick 'stress' and 'anger', for starters. You can probably also tick 'grief' and 'insomnia'. So keep reading.

Australians are getting better at acknowledging that mental health problems can happen to any of us, regardless of what job we do, how famous we are or are not, where we live and what our home life is like. However, we still have a way to go, before we realise that just because you can't *see* mental illness, this doesn't mean it isn't real – just because it's in your head, it doesn't mean though, that it's *all in your head* – if you know what I mean.

It's likely you don't consider that you have had or ever will have 'mental health issues'. But we've all had blue days. Or we know someone who has a lot of blue days. It's important to remember that these blue days are the result of a mechanical problem, the same as anything else that goes wrong with the body. It's a programming error and in a lot of cases there's a patch available.

Mental illness is one of the top ten leading causes of disease in Australia, with about 13 per cent of the total disease burden across the nation. Over the last three National Health Surveys (since 1995), the proportion of your fellow citizens with mental health issues has increased from 5.9 to 11 per cent. Some of that may be due to increased reporting rather than increased illness, but still . . . that's a lot of people. If you work in a company with ten people, that means statistically there's one person in your workplace with a mental illness.

Some interesting facts for you to know.

- Women are more likely to report high/very high levels of psychological distress than men (15 per cent compared to 10 per cent).
- High/very high levels of psychological distress were reported more frequently by adults who were separated (22 per cent) and divorced (18 per cent) than by adults who were married (9 per cent).
- The lowest rates of a high/very high level of psychological distress were among married men (9.4 per cent).
- Of adults reporting mental or behavioural problems in 2004–05, 32 per cent reported being current daily smokers compared with 20 per cent of those without mental behavioural problems.

It's also true that you have a higher risk of poor physical health if you do not manage any mental health problem you may have. Mental health problems can lead people to drink too much and do too little, take recreational drugs and smoke the cancer sticks in an effort to self-medicate.

The professionals

If you keep reading this chapter – or just dip into the bits you think apply to you – I'm hoping you'll learn when to ask for help before everything becomes too hard and too painful, and that you'll also learn where to go if you do need help or you need to help others. There is ALWAYS someone you can talk to, even if it's a stranger on the end of the phone.

In 2006 the federal government launched the 'Better Access to Mental Health Care Initiative' to make sure that services are in place for all of us. Those services are there for *you* paid by you with your taxpaying dollars. The initiative allows blokes like you to have subsidised consultations with your GP, psychiatrists, psychologists, social workers and occupational therapists regarding any mental health issue, for up to twelve consultations within a year. For many people who were previously unable to afford the help, this has opened up treatment options for the first time.

I realise that some of those professionals had some unappealing job titles, so let's demystify things a little bit.

- **General practitioner** – this is your 'local doctor', who is able to identify what you need and will either help you directly or refer you to a professional most suitable to help you.
- **Psychiatrist** – a specialised doctor who deals with mental health disorders. As doctors, these folks can prescribe medications and carry out medical tests or examinations. A psychiatrist, a.k.a. 'shrink' (short for 'head shrinker'), is not to be confused with a . . .
- **Psychologist** – a health professional who specialises in

dealing with the behaviours of individuals, the causes of those behaviours and their actions. Psychologists cannot prescribe medications. They may specialise in specific areas such as marriage and family counselling, drug addiction counselling, group counselling and child therapy.

- **Social worker** – a professional trained in problems specific to people and their family members, hence social workers in the community or in a hospital environment are there to help with social problems affecting issues revolving around every day life.

- **Occupational therapist** – a professional who provides assistance to those who find it difficult to cope with every-day tasks due to physical disabilities and mental health issues which limit the individual's work or social practices.

The parts

During one of my talks, a gentleman said to me, 'Stress is for losers. If you can't deal with stress, you're not a man. Some of these blokes these days need to grow some balls.' All his peers started laughing while completely changing their posture and putting on the 'I'm a bloke' face.

Yet at the end of the session, after everyone else had left the room, one of his colleagues came to speak to me to ask about ways of relaxing. He was finding work really hard to deal with, 'I feel like my body is permanently tense', he said. He explained that he felt his 'world was caving in, the little things are becoming bigger and bigger issues' for him to deal with. He had not spoken with his wife about these issues because he didn't want to worry her, as they had two young ones and a big mortgage. Leaving work or getting a job on the same money was unlikely, so it wasn't an option for him. I can only imagine how this bloke must have felt while his workmate sat there ranting and raving about what stress was.

Of course, it's possible that, for all his bluster, Mr Insensitive was actually covering up the fact that *he* didn't cope too well either. Why else would he feel the need to say something like that? No matter what front a person may put on, remember that you can never judge a book by its cover. Often it's the loud, attention-seeking individuals who are the ones unable to cope.

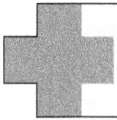

The 50 000 Km service

Let's take a look at the types of mental health issues that affect Australian men, so you can understand them a bit better.

- **Depression** is a state of unhappiness and the feeling of hopelessness. Along with this state of thinking, someone depressed may experience poor concentration, lack energy and contemplate ending his life.
- **Anxiety** is a feeling of nervousness and agitation, yet simultaneously a feeling of intense apprehension to carry out certain activities because of a sense of fear something will go wrong.
- **Bipolar disorder** – people with this condition experience the extremes of both manic (extremely elevated mood) and depressed (flat and sad) episodes. This can be distressing and extremely tiring for the sufferer and his friends and family.
- **Stress** is mental, emotional and physical strain due to either anxiety or too much work. Stress can impact heavily on

your health, causing high blood pressure and depression.
A little bit of stress can be a good thing – ask any physicist
– but ongoing stress is not.

- **Anger**, in clinical terms, is a very strong feeling of
annoyance. You just have to drive in a large city for half
an hour to see some fine examples of anger – otherwise
known as road rage. It is amazing who is willing to show
aggression over simple matters – road-ragers must have a
simmering stress level if they're so easily 'tipped over'.
- **Suicidal thoughts** means you are thinking of ending your
own life.
- **Insomnia** is the inability to get to sleep or sustain sleep.
- **Grief** is an intense sadness, sometimes indescribable in its
intensity. It usually follows the death of a loved one but also
occurs after any major loss, including losing a job or
a house.

Let's look at each of these in more detail.

Depression

Before you start saying, 'Nah, this section doesn't apply to me',
stop to think about some well-known public figures who have
recently confessed to suffering from depression. Men such as
Geoff Gallop, who resigned as Premier of Western Australia so he
could manage his illness; Brisbane Broncos player Justin Hodges,
English cricketer Marcus Trescothick, Australian cricketer
Andrew Symonds and former Newcastle Knights legend Andrew
Johns. Men about whom everyone said, 'I had no idea – they just
don't seem the type.'

Consider these facts.

- One in 5 people have depression at some point in their life.
- In Australia each year 1.1 million Australians suffer depression.
- One in 6 males are depressed.
- Twenty per cent of Aussie youngsters experience significant depressive symptoms.

  – *Taking Care of Yourself and Your Family, A Resource Book for Good Mental Health, Dr John Ashfield.*

Depression is a state of unhappiness and feeling of hopelessness which can affect your work and your everyday life. If this is the case, it is important to seek help. Depression can be an ongoing feeling for many – for weeks, months or years – often causing poor concentration, lack of energy and suicidal thoughts.

If someone has depression and keeps it to himself – not alerting loved ones or medical professionals – he will silently start to retreat into his own space, slowly saying no to various social functions he would normally never say no to and feeling a little estranged from those around him. Work becomes a pressure, even having dinner with friends becomes a burden. And taking responsibility for anything is a stretch.

It is really, *really* important to remember that depression is an illness, *not a choice*. Often there is no specific cause – it may just happen for no apparent reason. For many people this can be the most frustrating aspect of suffering depression.

Depression does not discriminate: it affects males, females, the poor, the rich, sportsmen, celebrities, mothers, fathers, brothers, sisters, uncles, aunts – even you. The good news is that while you can't choose to have the illness, you *can* choose to take steps to help yourself or others to prevent further progression of the condition.

There's no 'one size fits all'

There is not just one type of depression. You may have already heard of the following conditions:

- **Clinical depression** – this is also called 'major depression'. The sufferer's mood is very flat and may last for days, even weeks. It is often very difficult to lift a person from this mood without professional help.
- **Depression and anxiety** – an individual may be experiencing the two symptoms at the same time, feeling flat yet very anxious and nervous about their actions or what might happen.
- **Bipolar disorder** – this type of depression contains the extremes of high, manic moods and low, depressed moods. Some people find that in the high manic phase they can 'get a lot done' and 'have so much clarity', yet during the low phase 'it is almost impossible to drag your feet'.
- **Psychotic depression** – besides feeling depressed, there is also psychosis involved, where the individual may start to see or hear things or act in a rather peculiar manner, often coming across as paranoid.

CASE STUDY

During my third year of nursing studies I was sent to do a three-week placement in a psychiatric unit in Sydney. During my time there I met some very interesting people. The stories amazed me – these people whom others would have labelled as 'mad' were everyday people who had pushed their bodies and minds to their limits, resulting in mental illness.

I recall one man who was forty-four years of age; he was a local and owned a mechanics' shop just down the road. When I met this man he had been in the psych unit for three weeks, initially in the acute or high-risk section, which basically means he had the ability to be dangerous and cause harm to himself, the staff or those around him – this sort of patient is watched continuously by lots of nurses.

One day, in the moderate risk section, I sat and had lunch with this man. It was my second week, and it had taken this long to make conversation with this quietly spoken man.

I asked if he was feeling better, and when he thought he would be going home. He told me he felt very embarrassed about what had happened and was actually not very keen to face the people he loved the most.

'So what happened?' Looking back, that must have been the most intrusive, poorly timed question, but typical of a nosey student!

He swallowed and answered my question: 'I had a psychotic episode which, in all honesty, I cannot remember. I love to fish, you see, so one night I remember coming back from the beach with my rod and the next day I was in hospital. Apparently I strapped about five fishing knives to my body and walked out into the street yelling at people and threatening to cut the power pole down . . . Pretty silly, isn't it? My neighbours called the police and I was taken away.'

I asked if he had ever had that happen before. He said no, but went on to say he had been under considerable stress in the past six months, as his business was going broke and he just didn't know what to do about it – 'so I did nothing. It was just getting harder and harder, and I suppose I snapped, literally. But I'm on drugs now for my head, and I hope that makes it better, but I can't see myself leaving anytime soon.'

Apparently that was the longest conversation he had had with anyone in the three weeks he had been in hospital, so I felt quite honoured – but also felt such a sense of sadness for this man.

How would you know if your friend has depression?

Australians like to look out for their mates – and that means looking out for them in the bad times. Quite often depression creeps up on the sufferer, and the symptoms are more obvious to the people around him than to the sufferer himself. So it helps to know what to look for.

The common characteristics of depression are:

- Low self-esteem.
- Gradually spending less time with family and friends.
- Becoming moody at times.
- Being unusually sensitive to comments or jokes.
- Low libido (okay, you may not spot that one).
- Lack of intimacy (you may not spot that one either).
- Waking throughout the night or not being able to sleep.
- Becoming irritated by small things.
- Having less control over emotions.
- Using alcohol and/or drugs more frequently – if your mate goes from one schooner a day to half a bottle of whiskey, it's time to ask questions.
- Feeling tired a lot of the time.
- Tension or pain in the body.
- A tendency either to not be hungry or to completely overeat.

- Forgetfulness.
- A variation and fluctuation of feelings, from low in the morning to okay in the evening.
- Little motivation to do anything.

The triggers

Depression can affect any one of us, but there are certain triggers which seem to ignite depressive tendencies, such as:

Life stresses – these include changing jobs; separating from a long-term partner; losing a loved one; moving house; losing money on the stock exchange or your superannuation; divorce; being away from your children; renovating your home. Any one of these things can be stressful – and often people experience more than one of these at a time.

Having a long-term illness – according to Beyond Blue, long-term illnesses that are associated with depression include Parkinson's disease, epilepsy, diabetes, thyroid disorders, glandular fever, head injuries, heart problems (especially heart attacks) and cancer. It is also suggested that many of the treatments for these illnesses can also contribute to depression. The most important thing when dealing with long-term illness is to be honest about how you are feeling and let your doctor know if you are struggling emotionally.

Personality type can be a good indicator for those more at risk of depression. According to the Black Dog Institute, personalities at risk include those who are perfectionists, a little more self-focused, carrying high levels of anxiety, or those who appear a little reserved, almost shy, or who are self-critical. Sensitive individuals are also at risk.

Family history of depression – people are more susceptible to depression if their close relatives have had depression in the past.

Life-changing milestones adults reach can also be enough to cause depression. There are many thirty-year-olds going through a mini-life crisis, finding themselves speaking to counsellors because they haven't bought that house yet, haven't found the love of their life or their ideal job . . . They place all these expectations on themselves according to what they think *should* happen. Really, all they need to do is remove the word 'should' from their vocabularies.

There are the men going from Singleville to Marriedville, which can throw blokes out of their comfort zone, sometimes causing a feeling of loss for their old life. There are also many retiring from life-long employment to . . . What? Their living room? This can appear very daunting.

Depression becomes increasingly common in older people – think about coping with the loss of a loved one as you get older. The older you get, the more people you lose and it becomes harder to deal with. As Beyond Blue says, it is often difficult to assess older people with depression as the symptoms can be confused with dementia or forgetfulness. Not many people of the 'older generation' will tell you that they feel sad or down, and wrongfully we just assume that they will cope.

Gender also plays a big part in depression – while it is statistically proven that one in four women suffer from depression compared to one in six men, men are much less likely to seek help for feelings of loneliness or sadness, whereas women will speak to either their friends or professionals if there is something wrong. Possibly these statistics are not quite correct, simply due to the fact that women will be diagnosed whereas many men will not seek help at all. As Beyond Blue advises, if men were 'dealing' with depression, why is the suicide rate in men three times greater then it was back in the 1980s?

Living in remote country areas can also be a risk factor for depression. The feeling of isolation can sometimes be enough to contribute to a person feeling depressed. Compounding these feelings is the fact that people in these small communities often do not seek help, either due to not having the right professionals available locally (which is more often the reason), or not being able to afford the service. It also comes down to lack of privacy – can you imagine living in a town of just 800 people and worrying about being seen 'walking into the shrink's surgery' or 'people talking cause I'm on antidepressants and they'll see me pick up the tablets at the chemist'. These are real concerns. Real enough to stop people following up on health problems.

Sexuality is a huge issue for many men and women, boys and girls. According to Beyond Blue, people who are bisexual (attracted to both men and women) and homosexual (attracted to the same sex) are six times more likely to attempt suicide compared to heterosexual people (attracted to the opposite sex). The pressure for many homosexuals to 'fit in' – that is, be straight – can sometimes be too great, especially in smaller towns where acceptance may not be as great compared to a larger city.

Treating depression

There are various ways of treating depression – the treatment really depends on just how severe the depression is and what type of depression you might be experiencing. It is crucial that you get professional guidance to discuss treatment options – *do not even think* about treating yourself. Depression is not an illness that can be fixed by a few shots of bourbon each night, even if that seems to work at the time. As I said earlier, it's a programming error – and your doctor needs to help you fix the software. There is no shame in asking for help.

The options available range from simple lifestyle changes to quite long-term therapies. We'll look at some of them briefly.

Self-help and alternative therapies

There can be considerable benefit in using different or combined strategies, so when it comes to alternative therapies, you may need to use trial and error to work out what is most effective for you out of the following:

- Getting active.
- Good nutrition.
- Relaxation.
- Massage.
- Meditation.
- Aromatherapy.
- Vitamins.
- Herbs, eg. St John's wort.
- Light therapy.
- Alcohol free.
- Acupuncture.

- Drug free.

Here's a tip to spur you on . . . Serotonin, a naturally occurring chemical in the brain, affects mood, libido, appetite and sleep. Low levels of serotonin have been linked to depression. Research shows that regular exercise may increase levels of serotonin in the brain. Here's your simple feel-good equation:

Exercise = serotonin

Serotonin = improvement in mood

Ergo, exercise = improvement in mood

Psychological treatments

- Cognitive behavioural therapy (CBT) is a tool used by many therapists to help people realise what their thought processes are, showing the effect they can have on their mood. It may take six or more sessions for you to learn positive thought processes. There are some great CBT books available if you want to know more.
- Interpersonal therapy highlights certain social and personality factors which may also be contributing to your depression. The skills learnt should help you to identify certain depressive characteristics so you have the strategies and tools to help prevent you from experiencing further depression in the future.
- Psychotherapy can go on for many months or even years. The therapy allows you to discuss all of your history and then to slowly go back to specific situations to highlight how this is currently affecting you, helping you to resolve

these issues in order to move forward with your life, your actions and your thought processes. If you think this sounds like too much of a time commitment, stop and think about how long you've been feeling depressed.

- Counselling can be used to help with short- or long-term problems. It can give you strategies to help you get through specific situations, whether at home or in your workplace. Counselling can also be used in times of extreme situations, such as sudden loss of a loved one.

Drug therapies

These must be prescribed specifically for the individual and their condition. While the brand names change, there are some common generic names – these are the drugs most frequently prescribed in varying strengths, depending on the type of mental illness.

- Antidepressants
  - selective serotonin re-uptake inhibitors (SSRIs)
  - tricyclics (TCAs)
  - irreversible monoamine oxidase inhibitors (MAOIs)
- Tranquilisers
- Mood stabilisers
  - commonly used for bipolar disorder
  - lithium, valproate and carbamazepine
- Electroconvulsive therapy (ECT) – this type of therapy has had bad press from many years ago, but is still quite useful in various types of depression, such as:
  - life-threatening depression
  - severe mania
  - postnatal depression

Anxiety

Anxiety is a feeling of nervousness and agitation, yet at the same time there is intense apprehension to carry out certain activities in the fear something will go wrong. It affects up to 5 per cent of Australians. One in eight blokes will experience anxiety within any given year; one in four will experience it within their lifetime.

Anxiety can include feeling worried or concerned about a task you have to do, feeling unease or definite apprehension. It is quite common for all of us to feel pressure in life, and that's considered to be normal; but sometimes anxiety can affect your life on an everyday basis, and that is then seen to be a problem.

There are many different types of anxiety, including:

- Generalised anxiety disorder.
- Phobia.
- Obsessive compulsive disorder (OCD).
- Post-traumatic stress disorder (PTSD).
- Panic disorder.

Generalised anxiety disorder

This is a type of anxiety that seems to be ongoing, causing the sufferer to feel a level of anxiety every day, often worrying about everyday issues – things like home expenses, the kids or the car. This type of anxiety can, over time, cause you to feel restless, tired, tense and unable to concentrate, and you can have difficulties sleeping. So it can be fairly debilitating – in the 2004–2005 National Health Survey, 46 per cent of people with mental and behavioural problems had anxiety-related problems.

Phobia

This is when a person experiences a lot of fear towards a particular object, animal, activity or situation. To you or me the phobic's reaction may appear completely irrational, but the fear is so strong that it becomes uncontrollable and this becomes a mental illness that affects the person's life. Common phobias include:

- Acrophobia – fear of heights.
- Agoraphobia – fear of open or public places.
- Astraphobia – fear of lightning.
- Cenotophobia – fear of new things or new ideas.
- Claustrophobia – fear of enclosed places or spaces.
- Haemophobia – fear of blood.
- Mysophobia – fear of dirt and germs in places.
- Zoophobia – fear of animals.
- Xenophobia – dread of strangers.

Phobias are a little more common than you may think – up to 9 per cent of Australians suffer with them. It is entirely likely that one of your mates has a phobia – and no, not washing your underwear for two weeks doesn't mean you have a phobia of clean boxers.

Obsessive-compulsive disorder (OCD)

Also known as obsessive-compulsive behaviour, this can be cruelly dismissed as someone being 'anal retentive' or just plain 'frustrating'. Sufferers display obsessive behaviour over a particular task or thought process. A sufferer might feel compelled to tidy the house constantly or straighten a rug every time someone walks over it, or they constantly align each object in their home and the second someone comes along and disrupts this 'routine' they go into a total spin. Not only is it hard for the person who has OCD, as they are frequently feeling a high degree of anxiety, but for the partners or those around them it can also be really hard work.

Common OCD actions include:

- Continuously checking appliances to make sure you turned them all off the first time.
- Fear of touching public bathroom door handles.
- Fear of using dirty kitchen wear when out in public.
- Fear of having an accident or getting hurt.
- Constantly cleaning the house.
- Constantly washing hands or brushing teeth.
- Continuously needing order in the home, work, even in the car.

People with OCD can wash their hands until they are red raw or become so paralysed by their own behaviour that they can't work or leave the house. It's a serious illness – not just a funny little personality tic – so if you know someone with OCD, try to have a bit of sympathy . . . and also suggest they get some professional help.

Post-traumatic stress disorder (PTSD)

PTSD often occurs after someone has experienced a degree of trauma or shock, and can manifest as sudden, overwhelming anxiety, which can be extremely hard for sufferers to deal with. It is common to see PTSD in those who have served in war; have been involved in some kind of violence whether it be physical or emotional; have been in a major accident or rescued someone from an accident; or have seen sudden death. Even staying in hospital for a long period of time, with many procedures performed, can be enough to cause this type of stress disorder.

Those with PTSD have various experiences – it may just be simple flashbacks in the middle of work which cause the person to become very emotional, or they may experience trouble sleeping, have nightmares of the situation over and over again, feel a level of anxiety or find it hard to concentrate.

Panic disorder

This disorder, which includes panic attacks, is often a sudden onset of anxiety that is difficult to settle. It is only diagnosed as a disorder if a person has up to four attacks in the space of four weeks. Typical panic attacks will cause the person to be overly anxious, constantly fearing something is going to happen, and they may start to develop problems with their breathing. A panic attack can lead to people having chest pains, trembling and experiencing chills, feeling like they will be sick or the that they are going to faint. It can be a very intense, unpleasant experience.

How is anxiety treated?

Often the best form of treatment for anxiety disorders is psychotherapy. Psychotherapy can help you to recognise similar thought patterns or emotions which may trigger the anxious behaviour in the first place. This type of treatment allows you to change your thought processes and your reactions to similar circumstances in a more effective coping manner, in the hope of minimising any anxiety you might experience.

Psychotherapy includes:

- Cognitive behavioural therapy.

- Interpersonal therapy.
- Family therapy – family members and close friends are involved in the treatment to help guide the person to changing behavioural patterns but, more importantly, to educate those closest to the person about what type of anxiety the person has and what it can mean for the person.
- Psychodynamic psychotherapy – looking back into childhood circumstances which may impact on how the person deals with problems currently. This can be long-term treatment.

Then there are medications such as antidepressants and alternative therapies that will also help in cases of anxiety. According to Beyond Blue, some antidepressants can balance certain brain chemicals which often affect your mood, helping to minimise the effects of anxiety. Research indicates that when people have an anxiety disorder, specific changes occur in the brain chemicals – serotonin, noradrenaline and dopamine.

Where to go

Psychologists, psychotherapists and psychiatrists offer psychotherapy, but first see your GP so you can be referred to one of these specialists. You should see a specialist as soon as possible if your anxiety is severe, long lasting or could put you at risk of hurting yourself, or if the treatment you're on isn't really doing the trick.

If you think yourself or the person you are with is in a crisis situation – and this means that they're in danger of harming themselves or someone else – then you need to go to hospital. There is a 'crisis service' in most hospitals, or communities, which means people can come to you if you either can't go to the hospital or really don't want to go. Remember that you're not 'being a hassle' if you ask for services to help you manage a mental illness. An illness is an illness, and our medical services exist to treat illnesses. Call your local hospital or community health service.

In terms of alternative therapies which can help treat anxiety, think about:

- Exercising for a minimum of five days a week – this may sound like a lot, but it really works.
- Learning relaxation techniques.
- Trying to keep a balance in your life – not too much of anything, work or play.

We all have stuff that makes us anxious – the trick is knowing when you're feeling particularly vulnerable, so you can try to minimise anything that is going to cause you to feel a little anxious or on edge. For example, if you're working long days, your wife's just given birth to your first child and then you decide you're going to renovate on top of what is already going on in your life, you are potentially heading down the path to Stressville and then Anxiety Land – why do it to yourself? Slow down! Renovate later!

If you talk to any mental health professional, they will recommend you do the following when you're already feeling under pressure.

- Postpone big life changes.
- Address personal conflicts and aim to resolve them.
- Get some good-quality sleep.
- Do some fun stuff.

- Learn a little more about anxiety and helpful hints for managing it.
- Learn to say 'no' if you're a 'yes' person.
- Keep your work hours to a normal level – don't try to save the world.
- Seek help if you need it.
- Try to lay off the alcohol – it won't help you.
- Recreational drugs are a definite no-no.
- Be active – move it!

Bipolar disorder

Bipolar disorder is also known as manic depression and up to 600 000 Australians have it. The rate of alcoholism is three to six times higher in those with bipolar, and 30 per cent of patients referred by GPs to a psychiatrist, ostensibly due to depression, have bipolar tendencies.

Bipolar disorder involves extreme mood swings with the extremes of both manic (extremely elevated mood) and depressed (flat and sad) episodes, often caused by a chemical imbalance in the brain. This illness can be distressing for the individual affected and most certainly for their family and friends. Can you imagine what it's like being incredibly hyperactive – not able to sleep, not able to slow down – and then suddenly unable to cope with the idea of getting out of bed?

Bipolar disorder has managed to attract a lot of attention since rugby league player Andrew Johns announced he was suffering from the mental illness back in August 2007. If there was an upside to this, it was the fact that the media focus heightened awareness of the disorder – maybe it helped some people realise that they needed to get some medical attention for their own behaviour; maybe it helped family and friends of sufferers realise that their loved one isn't crazy, just unwell.

Andrew Johns has helped to change public perception about this illness and highlighted the need for more support and awareness in the community. I recall hearing a radio interview with Johns, in which he admitted, 'I thought the reaction to going public has been nothing but positive . . . I thought I'd be getting bars thrown at me and people taking the piss out of me, but it's been absolutely zero. Thought I would be getting slagged off in public, but there's been nothing . . . It's really surprised me'.

In October 2008, Johns promoted 'walk the walk' for bipolar disorder, a six-day trek from Newcastle to Sydney which created lots of media attention for the illness and the Black Dog Institute. He also had the support of many other Aussie personalities, including the prime minister, Kevin Rudd.

Although the reason Johns's illness first became public wasn't great – he was found with an ecstasy tablet in London – it did reveal an experience many bipolar sufferers have: self-medicating. If you suspect you have an illness like bipolar – if your mood swings are extreme, if you are manically up and then chronically down – please, please, PLEASE don't self-medicate. There are legal drugs that can help you – you don't need to drink lots of booze or smoke pot.

So what happens when you have bipolar disorder?

Let's have a look at the symptoms of the two different phases of bipolar disorder.

The Manic Phase	The Depressed Phase
Mood elevated	Feeling flat
Confident	Feel paranoid
Feeling sharp	Prefer to be alone
Sense of clarity	More sensitive than usual
Greater sex drive	Tendency to be quiet and
Super creative	reserved
Keen to spend more money	Fogginess with thoughts
Feel a sense of being 'high'	Do not feel as sharp or
Extremely happy	reactive
Wanting to laugh a lot more	Feel sad or down
than normal	May feel life is too hard
Become agitated	Suicidal thoughts
Impatient	Loss of confidence
Believe 'I can do anything'	Feel irritable

Who is more likely to have bipolar disorder?

There are several factors which can contribute to you getting bipolar disorder.

1. Genetics – you are 10 per cent likely to have bipolar disorder if one of your parents has it.

2. Health problems – poor health can be enough to trigger an episode and make changes to your 'normal' life very hard to deal with. The 'triggers' to watch for are:

- Thyroid disorders.
- Anxiety.
- Brain disorders or disease.
- Hormonal imbalances.

- Autoimmune disorders.
3. Lifestyle factors – extreme pressures due to:
  - Home life.
  - Losing a loved one.
  - Public scrutiny.
  - Work or changing employment.
  - Relationship dramas.
  - Divorce.

What's the treatment?

Treatments can vary for each person; most often a combination of treatments is recommended. Combination therapy is a mix of psychotherapy, drug therapies and 'alternative' or complementary therapies.

It's extremely important to use psychotherapy – such as cognitive behavioural therapy and family therapy – in combination with anti-manic medications such as sedatives or tranquilisers, mood stabiliser medications and antidepressants to help level out the highs and lows of the disorder. For some people, medications do not help. If this is the case, electroconvulsive therapy may be an option – and relax it's not like *One Flew Over the Cuckoo's Nest*. Electroconvulsive therapy now has a good reputation!

Relaxation techniques such as exercise are also very helpful. It may take some trial and error to figure out what works best for you – and once you know, it's crucial to stick to the strategies that help, such as exercising when you start to feel on edge, so you can go and burn off some excess energy before it becomes out of control. Maintaining a healthy lifestyle and balance can significantly help to keep your mental health at an optimum.

Initially it is important for the person affected to understand how the illness works, and this will help tailor the individual plan and also, hopefully, help the sufferer understand what may set off the mood swings in the first place – it could be a certain trigger, like alcohol. And as much as you may like your nights on the turps, they're really not worth it if they set off a manic episode.

If you or your mate or family member have bipolar disorder it's important to remember that it *can be controlled* with help and guidance from professionals who specialise in this area of mental illness. If you get that help, you can manage your life. If you don't, you'll keep suffering – which sort of life do you want?

Who should I see if I think I have bipolar disorder?

As with all mental illnesses, often the first professional to speak to is your doctor. They will ask you specific questions in order to assess whether you may or may not have bipolar disorder and will probably refer you to either a psychologist or psychiatrist.

It is also important to seek the support from those closest to you, whether it be family or a friend – often, just telling somebody you trust can take a very large load off your mind. I can't stress this hard enough: mental illness is nothing to be ashamed of. It's an illness like any other illness. The fact that you can't 'see' it doesn't mean it's not real and it doesn't mean you're not entitled to say that you have an illness. Also, because it's an illness, it can be treated. But, like the flu or heart disease or asthma, it can't be treated if you don't see a doctor or a therapist. You wouldn't expect to have an untreated heart disease and live a good life, because you can't – this is the same thing.

Stress

We hear the term 'stress' all the time these days – even little kids know about it – but what does it actually mean?

Stress is considered to be a mental, emotional and physical strain due to either anxiety or too much work. It can impact heavily on your health, causing various problems – most commonly high blood pressure and depression.

Stress affects people in numerous different ways – so much so that it can limit their everyday activities to the point where we now have stress leave provisions in the workplace – twenty years ago they were unheard of.

How do I know if I'm stressed?

Stress isn't a bad thing. In physics terms, stress is a force applied to an object in order to make it move. So stress is necessary – but **too much** stress is bad. According to the team at Beyond Blue the signs that you're too stressed are:

Difficulty getting to sleep	Feeling fatigued	Muscle pain
Difficulty staying asleep	Light-headedness	Forgetfulness
	Hard to concentrate	Feeling fearful
Feeling overwhelmed	Feeling anxious	Frequent urination
Shortness of breath while sitting	Low sex drive	Feeling anger or frustration
Muscle tension	Feeling dizzy	Having little appetite
Moodiness	Uncontrollable shaking	Heartburn
Nervous diarrhoea	Headaches or migraines	Feeling jumpy
Overreacting to things	Overuse of alcohol	Stomach cramps
Feeling nervous		

What types of things cause stress?

Let's start by saying that *everything* can cause stress. It all depends on the individual. You may find travelling to a foreign country stressful, yet your mates can't wait for the adventure. Jumping out of a plane can certainly be stressful, yet others may get off on the adrenaline rush.

Most commonly, the stressful events in everyday life are:

1. Moving house.
2. Changing jobs/careers.
3. Buying a house.
4. Selling a house.
5. Separating from a partner.
6. Working long hours.
7. Not enough time to see your family.
8. Divorce.
9. Losing a loved one.
10. Having kids.
11. Parenting.
12. Lack of support in the home, whether it be physical or emotional.
13. Driving in the city.
14. Leaving school.
15. Overanalysing situations.
16. Working with people.
17. Public speaking.
18. Working with computers.
19. Retiring.
20. Moving towns/countries.
21. Poor health.
22. Spending time with your wife.

23. Conflict with family/ colleagues/ friends.

24. Finances/debt.

25. Life-threatening illness.

26. Workplace conflict.

27. Ongoing pressure at work with minimal support.

28. Letting your kids go travelling.

29. Sitting exams.

30. Having an accident.

Another common form of stress is due to 'self-expectation' – that is, the expectations you impose on yourself about yourself.

If you have a family, you'd probably agree that you – and many of your mates – are concerned about putting food on the table for your family and providing them with all the things they need to live a happy and healthy life, along with wanting to protect them from all that is evil in today's world. That is a natural instinct in men, as is the need to be hardworking, to keep busy and skilled in what you do best. However, it's often these things that will cause you the most stress in your life if you do not have control over them – say, if you're made redundant or you have a workplace accident that lays you up for a while – or if you are not able to provide these things for your family or loved ones.

I think you'll find most blokes feel the same way at least once in their lives. As Dr Ashfield states in his book, *Taking Care of Yourself and Your Family*: '[T]his is important to understand in relation to men, whose roles make them especially susceptible to stress, because their brain and hormonal system are geared generally to the demands of action, productiveness, and exerting control over situations and environments.'

For some men, having to stay home to look after the kids

because your wife earns more money than you do, or the house is being repossessed, or you have been put off at work, are all major events that can cause you to become extremely stressed and possibly even depressed. Either of these states can have further consequences if you do not speak to someone and make positive changes in your life.

Remember: stress is *normal*. You're not letting yourself or anybody else down if you get some help to manage abnormal levels of stress.

Ongoing stress and your body

The following are very real symptoms of long-term stress. These are the red flags for your body, screaming for you to slow down and give yourself a break or there could be greater consequences. Don't ignore any of these if they pop up for weeks, rolling into months.

- Mouth ulcers.
- Stomach ulcers.
- Irritable bowel syndrome.
- Heartburn.
- High blood pressure.
- High blood glucose levels (which can affect diabetics, also causing weight gain).
- Skin rashes or irritations becoming increasingly worse.
- High cholesterol.
- Poor immune system – so you seem to catch every cold and flu going around.
- Muscle cramps and spasms.
- Inability to sleep.
- Feeling fatigued.

- Having anxiety.
- Continuously doing or thinking.
- Poor memory.
- Reliant on your evening tipple to help you relax.

And those dire consequences include:

- Cancer – it is believed that 'stress and destructive emotions can weaken or affect the body's surveillance system causing its immune response to fail to recognise and destroy cancerous cells' (Miller-Keane 1997 p.1540).
- Heart disease.
- Risk of stroke.
- Dependent on drugs and alcohol.

If you look at our society and the changes we have made due to the common mantra 'less time, need to achieve more', you'll notice that we have slowly let go of relaxation time. Whatever happened to Sunday being the day of rest? Sunday no longer stops. Every shop is open, every footy game seems to be crammed into the one day, and most people attempt to get everything done so they can start their week off again. At what point do you allow yourself to sit, read the paper, lie on your back under a tree or even go for a stroll?

When it comes to holidays and you get your four weeks off, it actually takes you the first two weeks to unwind and then the final two weeks to enjoy yourself. Too bad if your holiday is only two weeks long – or less.

I recall one night in the Cardiac Cath lab – we were called in to work at 11.30 p.m. to do an angioplasty on a 46-year-old man, a business owner, who was having a heart attack. Once the angioplasty procedure was done he told the staff, 'I don't have time for this, I've got to go on holidays in two days and there is too much to get done between now and then.' This guy was running on adrenaline, and had done for a very long time . . . No prizes for guessing why he was having a heart attack.

So what can I do?

The hardest part is working out that you are stressed – if you've made that step, well done.

The next step is to identify WHY you are stressed – what are the main causes? You may need to take a pen and a very large piece of paper to write down all the different things in your life that you think cause you stress. On the list will probably be:

- Home life.
- Relationships.
- Employment.
- Expectations you place on yourself.
- Perceived expectations others place on you.
- Goals.

Let's look a little more closely at how these may cause you to feel a bit stressed. And there's no judgement attached to this – don't judge *yourself* for getting stressed by this stuff, and don't judge others either. It's all part of life. The trick is not to get overly stressed.

Home life
- I have too many jobs to do around the house.
- The garden step I trip over every day on my way to work really shits me.

- Phone bills are too high – those bloody kids are always talking to their friends.
- The house is too small for five people.

As simple as these might sound, they all start to impact on one another, so after working all weekend around the house, waking up late Monday morning and tripping over the step as you leave for work can be enough to tick you off before you even begin your working week.

Relationships
- I feel like I'm always being told what to do.
- It feels like we're always fighting.
- I feel I can never do enough for her.
- Spending money we don't have on taking her out stresses me.
- We're not having sex like we used to – or at all.
- I'm questioning my sexuality.

Often relationship stresses are a result of poor communication, one small concern becomes increasingly larger, and more and more stressful the longer it continues.

Employment
- I'm working too much overtime each week.
- Nothing is ever organised.
- The boss doesn't communicate.
- Other blokes aren't pulling their weight and I end up doing all of it.
- My colleagues don't care about anyone else.
- There are unsafe practices in the workshop.

- I was promised more money, but they haven't talked about it since.
- I'm too busy, all of the time.
- We're expected to eat lunch at our desk – there's no time out unless you smoke.

Expectations you place on yourself
- I want a good car.
- I want to live in a big house.
- I'm a perfectionist, so I won't delegate anything to anyone.
- I want to get the promotion within the next twelve months.
- I need to work hard now to get my bonus at the end of the year.
- I want to pay the house off sooner.
- I want to buy an expensive engagement ring for my girlfriend.
- I need to be more dedicated at work.
- I want to keep others around me happy.

Some of these expectations may not seem much to you, but to other people they can be really stressful, causing the bloke to work harder or longer in order to achieve these things, often resulting in little balance and little happiness. Some of these things are often done to keep up an appearance for the sake of others – but, really, you're never going to know what other people are thinking about you, so why bother?

Perceived expectations from others
- They will think I can afford it.
- The boss thinks I want to be here for hours every night.

- My wife expects more from me.
- The kids really want to go to that private school, I can't disappoint them.
- They think I am the strong one – I can't show them how I'm really feeling.

This is what you *perceive* to be true, not what is necessarily true – unless you ask and gain confirmation from those you think feel this way, you are placing more stress on yourself then required.

I recall a colleague of mine working for a health organisation, performing medical checks on executives. One day a businessman was saying he was feeling quite stressed; he'd just had a high blood pressure reading. He started to talk about work being busy, but all five of his children were now going to a particular private school and the school fees were starting to affect the budget. He asked, 'How do you tell your kids you can't afford to send them to that school any more? They would be so disappointed in me, that isn't fair to them.' My colleague replied: 'It wouldn't be fair if they lost their father to a heart attack or to a mental illness, would it? They are kids, you don't need to go into the financials, but you need to be realistic to yourself and your wife. Don't try to keep up with the Joneses (whoever they are) – you have five kids, most others have two. Your expenses are a lot greater. Just do the right thing by your family and yourself.'

Goals and goal setting:
- I will have a deposit for a house in six months (if I don't do anything from now until then).
- I want the house to be finished in twelve weeks.

- I will be promoted this year.

Goal setting is important, but the goals need to be realistic and achievable, otherwise they too can become a stress.

It is important to actually sit and think about what really stresses you, so you can work out what you need to change to help lessen the load in your everyday life and make life generally less stressful.

When asking a few blokes what they do to relieve stress, the same answers kept cropping up.

- Have a cigarette.
- Go and do something physical in the shed.
- Go for a run or to the gym.
- Masturbate.
- Have sex.
- Yell at the kids.
- Punch the wall.
- Ride my motorbike.
- Yell and scream.
- Sit in my car and think it through.
- Eat.
- Go to the pub and get pissed.
- Go for a surf.

Some tips on avoiding certain stresses in your life.

1. Admit that you're feeling stressed.
2. Identify what is causing the stress, looking at all aspects of life.
3. Look at what you can change and be realistic.
4. Write a list and prioritise from most to least important.

5. Practise saying 'no' if you don't have the time to do something.

6. Look ahead at what you can do.

7. Take time, quit being in a rush all your life, it will wait for you.

8. Identify positive ways to relieve tension.

9. Practise relaxation techniques – make time each day for this.

10. Keep positive!

Anger

Anger is a very strong feeling of annoyance. Generally we think it's 'normal' for men to be the angry types, easily rising to the occasion of a fight or disagreement, because that's just what they do . . . Is it really, though?

Anger is just one of many emotions we all need to experience and certainly release. But not every day, in every situation. Let's look at the ways of dealing with and releasing anger effectively, rather than just bottling it up until you are ready to explode like a volcano – with more then just lava pouring out of your mouth.

Why is it important to release anger?

Often anger is the result of a whole bunch of other emotions you did not release when you probably should have. Let's say you're sad or disappointed about something, but instead of talking to anyone about it you go to the pub or just swallow your words, suppressing how you're feeling. It can be weeks, months, even years later when all the emotions explode. In the meantime, they've been festering away inside you.

Unexpressed anger will seriously affect your life and health in the long term. As the Men's Line Australia website says, it can cause:

- Tension throughout your body.
- Violence or aggression towards everyday issues.
- Aggression when drinking alcohol.
- Mental illnesses, depression, anxiety, insomnia.
- Troubled relationships.

Often it is a partner who may not understand why you are so angry all the time, or why you get angry when you drink. It's true that men find it very hard to express their emotions through words – 'I don't wanna talk about it, you won't understand', they might say. But often it's *you* who doesn't understand why you're angry. Anger can sit there for years – for something that happened when you were a kid – and it can rear its head without warning.

I should point out, however, that it's very important – and very difficult – to be angry with the right person at the right time for the right reason and in the right way. That's why you shouldn't blow your stack at your wife if you're actually angry at your boss. How can your wife change the situation with your boss? She can't. Get angry with the boss.

It's surprising what can build up over the years if you do not discuss the issues as they come to a head. One year just after Christmas (always the time for family feuds), I was out in a pub with family and as we were walking towards the restaurant, a group of twelve people walked in ready to sit down. As the group started sitting, a lady at the end of the table started yelling abuse. She threw the metal table number at her relative at the other end of the table, then stormed out crying hysterically. Next thing you know, other people started crying and half the group stood up and left, while the remaining few sat stunned. The moral of the story: take the person aside and discuss your issue, don't allow it to escalate to the point of no return. And remember to be angry *in the right way*.

How do I know if I have a problem with anger?

It can often be hard to realise you have a problem with anger when you're the one experiencing it. Maybe anger has become the norm for you – although you may start to question the reactions of those around you, and why they start looking at you like you're the one with the problem!

Ask yourself these questions.

- Have your friends or partner talked to you about your anger?
- Do you find you lose control over issues that really do not warrant it?
- Would you say you find it hard to control your aggression?
- Have you lost your temper to the point where you became violent towards those around you?
- Have you hurt somebody physically as a result of your anger?

If you have answered 'yes' to one or more of these questions, well, my friend, you may have an anger management problem. And it is a *problem*. Not a thing. Not an issue. A *problem*.

How do I manage it?

In order to manage anger, you first need to be aware of the onset of it and the feelings involved in order to recognise that frustration – a milder emotion – may actually be turning in to anger.

I love the analogy from the Men's Line Australia website: 'Anger is a car starting to roll down a hill. If you stop it quickly, it's relatively easy to bring it under control. If you wait until it's going at 60 km, it's clearly going to be a lot harder to stop.'

If you work in the public service, you probably know how easily people can become extremely aggressive over situations that are out of both yours and their control, yet somehow the aggression is thrown on to you for no other reason but you're the one who's there. Working in the hospital environment you often see a lot of anger coming from either patients or relatives, and admittedly it is often due to lack of communication or hours of waiting which really frustrates people (all of us, actually).

I recall an elderly man sitting by his wife during her stay in hospital. This particular lady was very ill and we had told the family to expect the worst. Now this elderly man could not speak English, so he was relying on his eldest son to explain exactly what was going on. During the family/medical meetings, we were unaware that the eldest son was not relaying a lot of the information to his father purely because he did not want to upset him, but, through lack of communication and frustration, and seeing the changes in body language from those around him, the patient's husband all of a sudden started screaming, kicking in the walls, punching the windows. It took three security guards to calm this man down enough to remove him from the unit. It is very difficult to reason with anyone once they become aggressive like this.

It is much better to deal with the feelings of frustration *before* they turn into anger. The first step is recognising the feelings you get before you start to feel angry. You may tense your muscles while you are talking, sweat may start to build under your shirt, or your face becomes flushed. Often your rate of breathing will increase, and there will be changes in blood pressure and heartrate.

Once I realise I'm getting angry, what do I do?

Basically, don't let the car roll down the hill – quickly grab a brick and chock it under the wheel and hold it right there.

At this point you can choose to either:

- Walk away from the situation.
- Remove yourself from the situation (once you have settled down, you can face the situation again).
- Calm down.
- Gather your thoughts.

The following tips can help.

- Practise deep breathing – take long, slow breaths until your breathing changes from fast and shallow to slow and deep.
- Practise self-talk – tell yourself 'relax or calm down, I can handle this'.
- Recognise triggers – are you drinking alcohol when this happens? Is it a particular individual who makes you angry? Is it losing a sporting match? Is it when you are upset with other relationships in your life?

How do I prevent myself getting angry?

As suggested by Men's Line Australia, if you do have excessive anger it is important to learn skills to avoid getting angry in the beginning.

You need to learn techniques such as:

- Conflict resolution.
- Communication.
- Relaxation.
- Changing certain beliefs about yourself or others.
- Anger management.

There is a list of websites and phone numbers at the end of the book, so please use these if you have any questions or concerns regarding you and your anger.

The emotional car crash – suicide

Any of the conditions or illnesses we've just talked about can make life very difficult to handle, and any one of them – especially depression – can make you think that life's really not worth living, especially since most people who commit suicide have an undiagnosed or untreated mental illness. Let's be really, really clear about this: *please*, it is worth doing *everything possible* to stop yourself from committing suicide. As a man, you are in a high-risk group for suicide – men are four times more likely than women to die from suicide, even though women commit more acts of self-harm than men.

Often people do not attempt suicide because they want to die – it's a form of escape from a situation or emotion that becomes too much to bear.

Quite often when a man commits suicide his family, friends and community say that 'he was always such a lovely bloke – who would ever have thought – he seemed to have it all together'.

Often they say this because the bloke who died did not discuss his problems. He tried to deal with everything on his own – and look where it got him. The suicide statistics reveal how difficult it is to cope with everything on your own. It's really difficult. Why do you think women talk to each other so much? Getting help – even if you think that people are going to think you're weak or whatever (and they won't) – is far preferable to leaving a life that still has potential. It's a better solution than leaving your family devastated and your kids' lives destroyed.

In today's current economic climate, with uncertainty and tough times ahead, suicide is even more of a concern. Blokes in the bush are killing themselves because so many years of drought have left them without viable businesses and they can't see a way out. Businessmen at the big end of town are killing themselves because they can't cope with the financial devastation. All of these men left behind families and friends who would, no doubt, much rather have done without the money than done without their mate or dad or husband.

The risk factors

You may never have thought about suicide. Or maybe you think about it occasionally. It can be something that just happens to you – a whole lot of things come crashing down. That's why you need to know what the risk factors are because you may not know you're at risk until you are. If any of the following apply to you, you need to be extra vigilant and *get help*. I'll say it again – GET HELP. TALK TO SOMEONE.

The most common risk factors are:

- Depression.
- Too much pressure felt at work.

- Financial distress.
- Loss of a loved one.
- Separation from a partner.
- Relationship problems.
- Unemployment.
- Dependence on alcohol or drugs.
- Previous suicidal tendencies.
- Trying to live up to family expectations.
- Isolating yourself from others.
- Ability to access guns, pills other potential suicide tools.
- You're extremely stressed, unable to cope with situations.
- Self-harming.

CASE STUDY

I once cared for a 24-year-old man who had attempted suicide in his home. His brother heard a noise and ran to the shed, to find the young man on the ground. Fortunately he survived. On questioning the young man, he admitted to attempting to end his life because he was set up in an arranged marriage and his parents had left the country to bring the young lady to Australia. This young man had a beautiful girlfriend but was told he 'must marry his own people' and the arrangement had been made for many years, therefore the family must keep their word or they would look like fools . . . This poor guy was so upset he thought there was no way out other than to end his life because he felt his parents and family would never understand.

On news of the son's attempt, the parents flew back to Australia immediately without the young lady. The parents explained to the staff that they only wanted their son to be happy and thought they were doing the best thing for him – 'but we want him to do what will make him most happy, we are so lucky he is still here'.

This young man couldn't see a way out of a situation he found unbearable but if he had talked about how he was feeling he may not have felt so alone and may not have seen suicide as a solution – as it turned out, his family were more understanding than he'd thought.

What could help to minimise the risk of a person committing suicide?

- Having a close relationship with family/friends.
- Being open and honest.
- A sense of purpose in life.
- Ability to problem solve and cope with life's ups and downs.
- Responsibility for others.
- Healthy attitude to life.
- Being social.
- Ability to talk to others when things get you down.
- A belief that suicide is not the answer.

The bottom line

If you are having suicidal thoughts please reach out and talk to someone. Your GP, your priest, a person at the end of a phone counselling line . . . there are people who can help you despite you thinking no one can. I am not making light of how you feel but trust me, suicide is not the ultimate answer to your problems – it is the ultimate non-answer. Once you're dead you'll never find out how much people love you and how much they could have helped you. Even if you genuinely feel that no one in your life would listen to you, there are professionals and counselling services who will. We are lucky to live in a country with a government that tries to take care of everyone – as much as the 'do-gooders' may drive you mad, sometimes they can help you too.

And if you are really, really set on the idea of suicide, ask yourself one last question: what if you'll feel better tomorrow? Or the day after that? Or next week? How can you be sure that things will *never* get better? Because they will. They always do. Particularly if you plan to make them better. You're the boss of you, and no one can change that. If you want to make a better life, there *will* be a way.

SOME USEFUL CONTACTS

- www.beyondblue.org.au
- www.blackdoginstitute.org.au
- www.mensline.org.au

Men's sheds

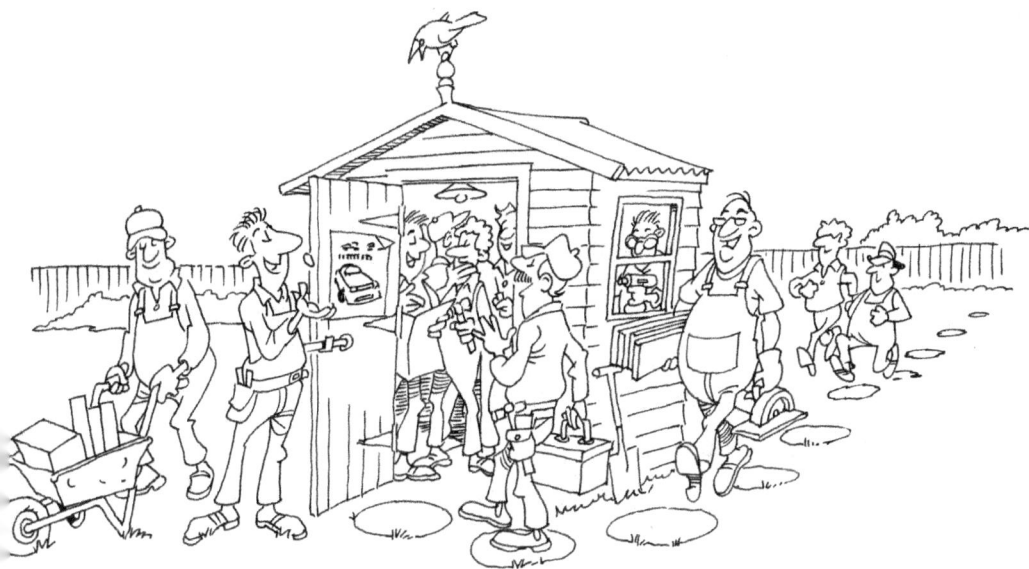

Men's sheds are starting to pop up all over the country, from large cities to small rural communities, in the hope of meeting the needs of men, improving their health and wellbeing, and their communities.

As the organisers say, 'All we need is a few good men'.

When I first heard about the idea of a 'men's shed' in various communities, I was keen to know more. After talking to the people involved, it was clear how much ongoing spirit and effort is involved in getting this off the ground.

Mensheds Australia is a not-for-profit organisation which started researching men's sheds in 2002. According to the organisation, at the time there were few men's sheds in Australia (maybe thirty), all operating under their own auspices. Mensheds Australia was established to help communities address the needs of starting, running and growing their own men's shed through out Australia.

The organisers say that the 'purpose of Mensheds Australia is to create an innovative approach to men's sheds development and help build sustainable men's sheds that are valuable assets for the communities they serve'.

The idea of men's sheds is to suit men's needs and wants, creating:

- A space for men.
- A daytime meeting place for men (not the pubs).
- Feelings of belonging.
- Social interaction.
- Reduced social isolation.
- Better addressing of men's health issues.
- Jobs and business opportunities.
- Improved lifestyles leading to improved quality of life.

Fundamentally, too, the sheds give men their lives back and build better communities.

According to Mensheds organisers, a men's shed can go a long way in assisting men to cope with the three big health issues of isolation, loneliness and depression.

Many sheds differ in their focus but they all relate to the men's needs and the needs of the community. Some of the sheds work on specific projects, such as restoring bicycles to give to disadvantaged kids or communities; others make furniture to be sold for both charity and the upkeep of the shed. Sometimes there are guest speakers who come along to give a talk on various health issues affecting men's health. One community has built men's-only accommodation for those going through financial difficulties or separation, giving the men in the community a place to get back on their feet with the support of their peers.

In Titjikala in the Northern Territory, the local men have started a men's shed without the shed. The aim for these guys is to improve the physical and mental health of the local community members. According to Mensheds Australia, the 'health of indigenous men is significantly worse than for any other group in Australia, with an average life expectancy of only fifty-nine years – some twenty years less than non-indigenous Australian males. Indigenous men often have to contend with many barriers to improving their health, establishing businesses, employment and training and therefore require additional assistance in order to gain access to the same opportunities as non-indigenous men. Men are men, no matter where they are, and they all seem to suffer from similar issues.'

Often men reach retirement and sit at home after the first twelve months wondering what use they are to society, and this causes an element of depression and unhappiness in their lives. The men's shed movement helps men discover or rediscover an interest, allowing them to use their brains and their skills while teaching others new skills, to help carry these through the community for generations to come.

Recently there was an article about the men's shed in Parkes, NSW, where a few of the men's wives would call in at 10 a.m. on set days to bring the men some scones and make them cups of coffee and tea, giving many locals something to look forward to. One of the wives interviewed said, 'I have seen such a difference in my husband since he's been coming down to the shed three days a week. We now have something to talk about when he comes home, and it gives me some time to myself too. I think it's a great idea. My husband is not the type to play golf or go to the club, so what else is he going to do if you don't have other interests?'

This is exactly the essence of a men's shed. What do men do if they do not have an outlet once they are retired, or even before they are retired? Men do not necessarily want to sit in a club half their day with mates – many are more then happy to be standing around in their shed, chatting away while working on small jobs.

The face of Mensheds Australia is a bloke by the name of Col. Apparently 'Col is the epitome of the Aussie mate who is always ready to lend a hand and if you really needed a mate he would be there. His willingness to pass on his life skills makes him a role model for the youth of today.' This is what our society needs to be reminded of. It is the small things in life that are often much more important then anything else we think we might need – 'true, genuine mates'.

How will men's sheds affect men's health?

When I look at ideas of promoting men's health, I'm looking at how best to deal with getting the message out there and what angle is needed to raise awareness. However, as Mensheds Australia points out, 'It is pointless trying to do anything without engaging the men to work on their own problems'.

Mensheds Australia believe isolation and lack of identity among men in rural and remote areas are major issues, so the idea of a shed where blokes can congregate for multiple reasons may just indirectly help to address these issues and have a longer-lasting affect on both the morbidity and mortality rates of our Aussie blokes. We only have to see the statistics on suicide to know that we have a significant problem.

The team at Mensheds Australia agrees that the main problems within the communities range from isolation, unemployment, mental and physical disabilities to loneliness, depression and alcohol abuse.

The idea of men's sheds throughout the country is to help minimise the risk of men feeling isolated or lonely, especially once their working life comes to an end, often resulting in depression and further health problems as a result.

If men know there is a life after retirement, or ways in which they can help their community – and projects where their skills are needed, no matter what they might be – it will help open up the lives of those who thought the doors were already starting to close.

Men's sheds are springing up all over Australia and are being recognised by health professionals and governments as a significant catalyst for improving the lives of men. As Peter Sergeant of Mensheds Australia says, 'it is an idea whose time has come'.

SOME USEFUL CONTACTS

Contact the guys at Mensheds Australia to find out where your nearest men's shed is to you or if you are keen to get a shed up and running in your local community on (02) 8213 8699 or www.mensheds.com.au

You are what you eat

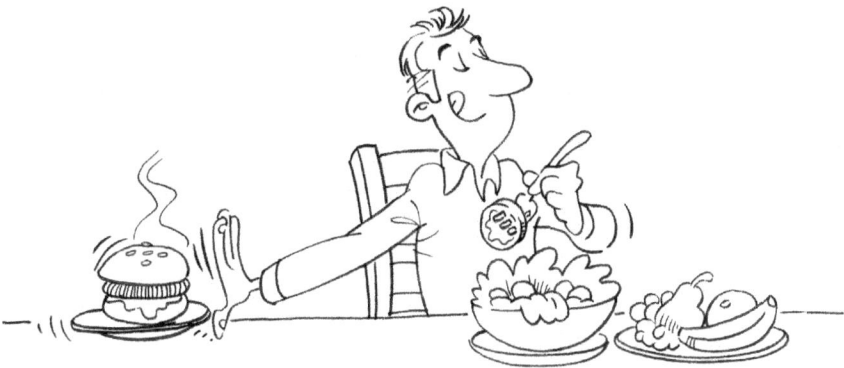

You wouldn't put watered-down petrol into the tank of your beloved maroon Nissan Skyline, would you? Nor would you use fish oil instead of motor oil, liquid drainer instead of radiator fluid, or your kid's Nintendo Wii instead of a battery. You have to use the good stuff to get the best performance out of your vehicle. The human body is exactly the same. (For those of you in IT land, here's an old computer analogy: garbage in, garbage out.)

In my work as a nutritionist I often meet people who run their lives on foods similar to 'dirty' petrol – then they wonder why they can barely make it up the hill. Frustratingly, when I give these people a few nudges in the right direction of a better fuel station with good quality fuel, they whinge and tell me it's too expensive . . . Well, lads, you get what you pay for! So the dirty fuel becomes the habit, the easy option, and I guess their attitude is that if they've always run on the poor quality stuff, they won't really notice the difference if they don't change it now. To that, I say: WRONG.

We all know what happens to cars that aren't taken care of. They break down regularly, usually with expensive results. All a car needs to run for years is a twice-yearly service and the right fuel (plus the odd spit and polish), and all that is far cheaper than fixing it up once it's broken down. Not to mention the fact that a broken-down car usually requires roadside assistance from your friendly state organisation, plus a tow truck, plus a whole lot of swearing on your part and a world of inconvenience. And all because you couldn't be bothered taking it round the corner for a service . . . So why is it hard to believe that choosing the slightly more expensive fruit and vegetables over meat pies and ice cream works out to be cheaper – and less painful and inconvenient – in the long run than having a quadruple bypass operation, with all the time off work and radical lifestyle changes that go along with it? *Why would you treat your car better than you treat yourself?* It's no use having a smooth ride if you're too unwell to drive it.

I've decided that, rather than being wilfully badly nourished, most blokes eat badly because they don't know any better. Sure, in the deep, dark mists of your childhoods you knew about bananas and boiled eggs and three veg for dinner. But once you hit the teenage years and your habits went awry, it was hard to find your way back. It's a bit like loving the Rolling Stones as a little tacker and then deviating to Cliff Richard – or, heaven help you, Ricky Martin – because you liked that one song he had that one time . . .

The good news is that there is always a way back to Mick and Keith. And I'm here to tell you what it is.

The short description

Nutrition is not just about 'Chocolate is bad and fruit is good'. Nutrition looks at the science of foods, the nutrients which make up foods and the effects they can have on the body, both good and bad. Nutritionists look at all spectrums of the body when we assess a person's nutrition, including when they eat the food; how they digest the food; their absorption of certain foods; how food is carried throughout the body, from the stomach to the bowel, and how long it takes for your body to break food down (metabolise) in order to benefit from it. Last but not least, we consider the waste products, otherwise known as urine and faeces – what your body cannot use it very efficiently gets rid of!

The main reason we eat food – besides the fact we might *like* food – is to supply our bodies with nutrients, and plenty of them. Nutrients and essential nutrients (nutrients our bodies can't live without) are otherwise known as great energy sources. Even a seven-year-old could tell us the daily foods and nutrients our bodies need – carbohydrates, proteins, lipids or fats, vitamins and minerals and, obviously, we need water.

These types of foods and nutrients are essential to enable us to grow, repair, heal and maintain our everyday functions. Ideally we should eat what our bodies can use: high nutrient-dense foods (vegetables, fruits, quality proteins and good oils) along with drinking lots of water (1.5 to 2 litres) during the day.

My motto is: Aim to eat what your body can use. Otherwise, if you can't use it, lose it!

While you're reading this chapter, instead of thinking, 'Gah, how boring!' when I talk about eating bananas instead of burgers, take the time to think about how you actually feel after eating certain foods. It's the only way you'll get to know what your body enjoys and which foods it benefits from. Sure, junk food makes your tastebuds feel good while you're eating it, but it's a temporary joy. Afterwards your stomach, gut and bowels will *not* be happy about it and you'll feel like crap. Yes, sirree – crap. Never let it be said that I don't give it to you straight.

The parts

Let's talk about all the good stuff you need to eat. We'll start with protein, since that's been in the news a bit lately. Atkins this, CSIRO that.

Protein

We all need to eat protein daily. We don't need a lot of it, but we do need it every day, and if possible it's best to have the good-quality stuff. Many people I chat to associate protein with a good-sized quality steak, but this isn't true at all. The grains we eat are a high protein-rich food source. I know – *some* of you are vegetarians. Maybe even vegans. I'm an equal-opportunity nutritionist. Which is why I'm going to tell you that there are two types of proteins.

Animal proteins include meats, poultry, eggs, fish and seafood, milk and dairy products. These are considered to be the best source of protein, containing all the essential amino acids. These amino acids are very important for maintaining our muscles, immune system and cells.

Plant proteins include grains, legumes (beans, chickpeas, lentils), nuts and seeds. These are considered 'incomplete' proteins as they lack one or more amino acids so if you combine many of these types of foods, they will be a 'complete protein'. Examples of these combinations include:

- curried dahl with rice.
- hazelnut spread on wholegrain toast.
- porridge with nuts and seeds.
- chickpea salad with quinoa.

Why bother eating proteins?

Your body uses protein in a variety of ways, which is why it is considered an important food. Just some of the reasons you need protein include:

- Your body's growth.
- To transport oxygen from your lungs to tissues via your blood.
- It helps keep your iron stores within normal levels.
- It helps transport vitamins and minerals around the body.
- It boosts your immune system, protecting the body against disease.

- To provide your body with energy.
- It helps to regulate your metabolic rate – this is very important when it comes to maintaining your weight.
- To regulate your fluid and electrolyte balance.
- To maintain the function of nerves, hormones and muscle.
- To regulate body fluid pH (keeping acid levels within normal ranges).

Basically, if your body does not have sufficient protein, the many body functions we take for granted, as highlighted above, simply would not happen.

How much protein should you be eating each day?

It is recommended that a person eats 0.8 to 1 gram of protein per kilogram of body weight daily. What many people – menfolk included – do not realise is that this recommended amount is the *actual amount of protein* you should be eating, not the weight of the food that contains the protein. Actual protein in a food differs from the weight of that food. For example, a piece of fish weighing approximately 110 g will contain approximately 29 g of actual protein.

To illustrate (and to flex your maths muscles): a bloke – let's call him Jim – is a 100 kg forklift driver and he's come to see me. How much protein do you think I should recommend that he eats? At Jim's weight, he should be eating around 80 g to 100 g of actual protein per day. Jim can find this amount of actual protein in protein-based foods such as nuts, lentils, eggs and meat. It's ideal to eat this total amount over the course of the day but not in one sitting – although for some reason people often laugh at me when I say this . . . It's true, though: a 300 g steak is just too much for your body to absorb at once.

As I'm enjoying the maths of all this – and because the concept can be a wee bit hard to grasp at first – let's look at some examples of how much actual protein is in different types of foods that you probably eat.

425 g can of tuna	=	93.5 g of protein
1 large boiled egg	=	6.6 g of protein
50 g (small handful) raw almonds	=	10 g of protein
50 g brazil nuts	=	7.2 g of protein
200 g chicken	=	62 g of protein
200 g beef (lean fillet)	=	64 g of protein

In case you don't want to take this book to the local grocer when you're buying food you can check the 'food label' panel on the side of your food – look for the **PROTEIN** section. There's also a very user-friendly website called Calorie King: www.calorieking.com.au.

Sinking the protein ship

It is possible to eat too much protein, and this can be a bad thing. Health professionals can't agree on whether excess protein consumption or high saturated-fat food is the real culprit for causing the following:

- Heart disease.
- Cancer.
- Osteoporosis.
- Weight control and obesity.
- Kidney disease.

If you're consuming protein powder or drinking protein shakes – and a lot of men do this if they're working out at the gym a lot – you'll need to make sure that you don't exceed that recommended rate of protein intake. Don't forget to include the protein powder or shake in your daily protein tally. And remember when it comes to your body, it's more about the quality of the protein you are eating, so don't go cheap, buy yourself quality, not quantity.

Carbs, carbs, carbs

Well, haven't these been given a bad rap lately? Carbohydrates seem to be everywhere, in all different shapes and sizes, and some people think all of them are bad. They're not all bad, and anyway, it's all in how you eat them.

Some carbs (let's just call them that, since everyone else seems to) are the equivalent of your Commodore (settle down, Ford drivers!) – they help you run around and get things done, and they're just bloody everywhere. Bread would be the carb version of the Commodore.

Other carbs are like an Aston Martin – they're not seen often and only then with people who can really afford them. Most people have to work them off for too long as opposed to pay them off, remember often these machines look better then they actually drive, so is it worth it?

Sweets would be your Aston Martin.

And some carbohydrates – the most useful carbs – are like your Toyota Hi-lux: you can depend on them every day, and they'll help your body stay fit and healthy (because you're hauling things on and off the tray).

Carbohydrates are certainly required in our every day diet, but there are good and bad carbohydrates we can choose to eat. You have to choose your carbohydrates wisely if you want overall health and happiness. Lots of Hi-lux, a liberal dose of Commodore and very little Aston Martin.

What are carbs?

Carbohydrates come predominantly from plant derived foods (and yes, fruit and vegies are carb foods, due to the fact they release glucose slowly into the blood stream, along with an amount of fibre. These little beauties are worth much more praise then we give them).

- Grains and cereals.
- Vegetables.
- Fruit.
- Legumes.
- Nuts and seeds.
- Sugar.
- Honey.
- Refined foods.
- Milk and other dairy products.

These foods – except the sugar – will contain other nutrients (vitamins and minerals) which are helpful to your body.

What do carbohydrates do for your body?

- They're a great source of energy – helping to keep our brains and bodies functioning.
- They supply glucose to your body's cells to produce energy.
- If you eat excessive amounts of carbohydrates, your body

stores it for later, in case you need it. It is like it knows what happens, when you're waiting in a long queue for pies at a Richmond game and you're convinced the last quarter will have started by the time you get a pie – and you started queuing at kick-off.

- They're a great source of fibre.
- Important for the digestive system.
- Help to reduce fats and glucose in the bloodstream.
- Reduce the risk of obesity /heart disease /cancer /diabetes / gut problems.
- After you've eaten a meal containing carbohydrates the level of glucose in your bloodstream (blood glucose) will increase, stimulating the release of the hormone insulin. Insulin stimulates the uptake of glucose from the bloodstream into tissue cells. Consequently if excess glucose is eaten and you do not do enough activity to use it, it will be stored, later converting to fat.

I had a client tell me whenever he is eating anything white in the carbohydrate family it gives him a sedative effect – he 'just needs to lie down for twenty minutes'. The foods he was referring to were white bread/rolls and large pasta dishes and they can cause a spike in the blood glucose level (due to a high amount of glucose entering the bloodstream).

The client was feeling extremely tired after eating white bread because he later found out he had the onset of diabetes. While the glucose was being released from the food he was eating, the insulin wasn't travelling fast enough and was only picking up half of its usual load of glucose. The client needed to start eating better forms of carbohydrate that released sugar into the blood slowly and he also needed to go onto some medication to help the insulin do its work.

White breads can certainly have this effect on some people and yet not on others – it's all about learning what is right for you and what your body feels happy with.

How much carbohydrate should you eat?

Australia's National Health and Medical Research Council (NHMRC) has not implemented a recommended daily intake (RDI) for carbohydrates as your daily intake really depends on the amount of activity you perform each day.

The Australian Guide to Healthy Eating recommends at least four to seven servings of breads and cereals every day for the average individual.

Serving size varies on the type of food. According to Jennie Brand-Miller, one of Australia's leading dieticians and nutritionists:

1 serve of a carbohydrate-based food is:
- 2 slices of bread
- 1 corn cob
- ½ cup oats/muesli
- 1 cup breakfast cereal
- ½ cup cooked rice/smaller grains
- 1 cup cooked pasta, noodles or couscous
- 2 small potatoes or half a medium sweet potato

1 serve of vegetables is considered to be:
- ½ cup cooked vegetables
- 1 cup raw/salad vegetables

- 1 cup vegetable soup or juice

1 serve of fruit is considered to be:
- 1 medium piece or 2 small pieces
- 1 ½ tablespoons sultanas
- 4–5 apricots/figs/prunes
- ½ cup fruit juice

Too much of a good thing

As mentioned earlier, carbohydrates are required for our energy levels, but if you consume more carbs than can be used by your body (by being physically active) this can have a few effects, primarily:

- Weight gain – remember, carbohydrates break down into glucose, helping supply the body's cells with energy, but if too much energy is consumed and not used through being active, the glucose will be stored for later . . . and if it's still not used later, it's stored as fat. Weight gain will and can then predispose you to further health-related problems, as I'm sure you already know.
- Altered blood glucose levels – the release of glucose into the bloodstream is raised, therefore greater amounts of insulin are required in order to pick up the glucose within the blood, to help normalise the blood glucose level.

Lipids/fats

Lipids – better known as fats (but 'lipids' sounds better, don't you think?) – are the types of nutrients we 'use' when we have to. However, we shouldn't consume them too often. You may have them every day, but just briefly – just enough to keep you happy, such as butter on toast. Note that buttered toast should be consumed in moderation.

If you start using fats everyday in too many ways, you'll start to pick up extra calories because your body won't be able to use that much fat. So the unused fat will be stored as love handles a.k.a. the dreaded spare tyre, and before you know it, you're a fatty. So, like all good things, a little bit of fat goes a long way. This means having a little bit of brie, not the whole wheel.

It's also important to know that some fats are bad and some are good. So we're gonna break it down for you.

Lipids means triglycerides (fats and oils), phospholipids and sterols.

Fats contain mostly triglycerides and are found in both foods and the body.

Oils are liquid fats at room temperature, such as olive oil.

Saturated fat – is a type of fat that can be harder to break down in our body, often raising the blood cholesterol level. Saturated fats include meats with visible fats (such as marbled meat), coconuts, coconut and palm oil or palm kernel oil, commercial cake, biscuits, takeaway meals, potato chips, dairy products – cream, cheese, milk, butter, yoghurt, lard. If this describes the sum total of your daily diet, you need to be afraid. Very afraid. (A little exception: coconut oil is a saturated fat but it is still considered a safe fat to heat and cook with as it can endure high levels of heat).

Monounsaturated fat is made up of triglycerides, while missing two carbon atoms from the saturated fatty acid chain. Examples include olives, vegetable oils, margarines and some nuts.

Polyunsaturated fat is made up of triglycerides where most of the fatty acids are considered to be polyunsaturated. What this means is they are lacking in more then two carbon atoms and hydrogen atoms. Examples include fish oils, sunflower and sesame seeds, vegetable oils (sunflower, flaxseed, sesame oils), safflower oils, corn oil, soybean oil, cottonseed oil and some nuts are polyunsatured fats.

Cold pressed are the better choice when cooking with oil. The olive is pressed within normal conditions with minimal heat used, in order to extract the oil from the olive. A process that is much safer for your body when using the cold-pressed oil.

Hydrogenated fat is the fat that develops when we choose to cook with or heat a monounsaturated (olive oil) or polyunsaturated (vegetable oil) fat (like in deep-fried and baked foods). This may sound over-the-top but bear with me. The heating process causes hydrogen to attach to the chemical structure of the fat, making it much harder to break down, consequently changing the fat from a monounsaturated/ polyunsaturated fat to a solid form, resulting in a trans fat.

Trans fat fats are much harder for the body to break down due to their complex molecular structure. A great example of how the trans fat develops can be seen in your local fast food store. It is on the hot chips you buy, where the oil sitting in the fryer is continuously heated and cooked over and over again throughout the day and in most cases re-used for weeks, in order to fry the chips within minutes. Once we reheat oil that has already been heated in order to become liquid, we are changing its chemical structure, which makes it more difficult for the body to break it down. This process causes cholesterol (plaque) to remain in our blood vessels. Trans fats are dangerous for your health!

Cholesterol is found in your blood and considered to be a fatty substance. Cholesterol is required for our everyday bodily functions, but if the levels of cholesterol in our blood become too high it can be detrimental to our health. We have 'good' (HDL or high density lipoproteins) and 'bad' (LDL or low density lipoproteins) cholesterol in our blood.

The good oil on fats

Different types of fats play specific roles within the body, all with varying health benefits.

Monounsaturated fats are believed to reduce cholesterol levels, helping to reduce the risk of heart disease. Great food sources include avocado, raw nuts (e.g. almonds, peanuts and cashews), monounsaturated margarine, peanut oil, olive oil and canola oil.

Polyunsaturated fats help lower blood cholesterol levels. These fats involve fatty acids such as the commonly known Omega 3 and Omega 6. Omega 3 and Omega 6 fatty acids are important for our immune, cardiovascular, nervous and neurological systems, and vision.

Omega 3 foods include oily fish (salmon, sardines and tuna), flaxseed oil, fish oil, poultry, walnuts and pumpkin seeds. Omega 3 is mostly considered healthy for helping lower the 'bad' (LDL) cholesterol levels and along with it the risk of heart disease; depression, and premature birth. You will certainly see the value of EPA (eicosapentaenoic acid) and DHA (docosahexaenoic acid) on the sides of salmon or tuna cans and fish oil capsules or liquid, so look at the label to find out.

Omega 6 foods include poultry, sunflower oil, soybean oil, some margarines and nuts. These fatty acids help in lowering total cholesterol.

The bad oil on fats

Let's make it simple, fats are necessary, but again, it's all about the quality and the quantity, if you eat too much or eat poor quality food you are going to end up looking at possible:

- Heart disease.
- High blood pressure.
- Cancer.
- Obesity.

I've never met anyone who actually wants to have any of these illnesses. Next time you consider eating a block of cheese or three Big Macs in one sitting, ask yourself why you *want* to have one of those illnesses. The answer I usually hear for over-eating – 'Because cheese/meat/etc is delicious' – isn't really that convincing.

What should your cholesterol levels be?

The recommended levels are:

- Total cholesterol – <5.5 mmol/L
- LDL – <3.5 mmol/L
- HDL – >1.2 mmol/L
- Ratio of LDL: HDL – <3.5:1

This actually won't mean anything unless your doctor takes you through it. Cholesterol levels can be moderated through diet and, if necessary, medication but you need to do it in consultation with a medical professional. Although a lot of blokes seem to think 'She'll be right, mate' applies to most health matters that don't affect their ability to play their favourite sport, your cholesterol levels could end up affecting your ability to even watch your favourite sport. Cholesterol levels can be an indicating factor, but don't be fooled – you can still have low cholesterol levels and have heart disease! Remember it is your HDLs you want to increase!

What a doctor talks about when they talk about cholesterol

When – not *if* – you visit your doctor for a cholesterol check, you'll be told about the following:

Total cholesterol takes into account the combination of the LDL and HDL within your blood.

The LDL (low density lipoproteins) level refers to the amount of 'bad' cholesterol in the blood. The role of LDL is to *deliver* cholesterol to different tissues of the body, so if there is excess cholesterol it accumulates in the arteries, causing potential damage. This is why it can be 'bad' cholesterol.

The HDL (high density lipoproteins) level refers to the amount of 'good' cholesterol in the blood. The HDL mainly *removes* cholesterol from the tissues of the body, transporting it to the liver, lowering cholesterol being deposited in the arteries.

The LDL: HDL ratio refers to how much of one is present compared to the other within the total cholesterol level.

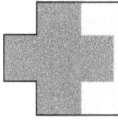

The 50 000 km service

Lots of us struggle with our weight. And – there's no nice way to say this – being overweight *always* adversely affects your health, whether it increases your risk of getting heart disease, diabetes or cancer, or it exacerbates an existing condition. Sure, getting fat is fun – you eat all that food, you laze around and don't do any exercise. But being a fatty is *not* fun.

Becoming a fatty is not as simple as eating too much and not exercising enough – although they're the main culprits. Your metabolic rate has a role to play, as does fatigue. And then it all seems too hard to lose weight. Being a fatty seems easier.

Let's put it this way. Your body is like a racing car (I'll let you pick the make and model). Racing cars are designed to perform optimally *if* they are handled properly. Let's say the car sits in the garage and you keep loading it up with gear because you know it's not leaving the garage anytime soon. You leave clothes on the back seats; you load up the boot with containers of oil and old tools. That car gets heavier and if you tried to drive it you'd be placing an amount of pressure on the motor, chassis and tyres. You'd be on the road thinking that the racing car is not so racy and then you'd take it back to the garage and leave it there, knowing that it's never going to win any kind of competition. Eventually you'll blame the car for underperforming and probably sell it.

However, if you kept that car in motion – if you took it for a burn around the track on a regular basis, kept the junk out of the boot and made sure that it had the right fuel and a regular service – that would be one happy vehicle. Everything would work properly because it would be doing what it was designed to do. Your body really isn't any different.

For those of you more mathematically than motoring inclined, let's look at the following equation to explain weight gain and loss:

Energy in vs Energy out

Loads of food (calories) in and little movement of thy butt = weight gain.

Little food (calories) in and lots of movement of thy butt = weight loss.

Same amounts of food (calories) consumed as energy (calories) used = no weight change.

Get a'sweating!!!

The slow build

It's often the little things we do on a daily basis that contribute to the weight piling on, so it happens slowly over time, although it seems like the flabby parts have suddenly materialised with no warning. Have a think about what you do on a daily basis that may put on weight slowly. It could be:

- Upsizing meals, so not only will you eat a burger and chips, you will have the extra-large version, adding almost more than double the amount of energy into your belly then you needed.
- Drinking three large coffees every day, each of them containing milk and sugar.
- Grabbing a quick croissant every morning at the bakery on the way to work.
- Drinking two litres of soft drink every day.
- Living on takeaway meals because it's quicker when you work such long days.
- Eating hot chips every lunchtime at work.
- Grabbing a Chico roll for morning tea.
- Opening a pack of nuts to nibble on while you cook dinner, then finishing the entire bag by yourself (within twenty minutes).
- Having a second plate of food every night after dinner.
- Drinking four or five alcohol-based drinks every night.

Avoiding the slow build

Clearly it's better to avoid falling into these traps if you can – I know, I know, it's easier said than done. Truthfully, though, it's easy done too. *Really*. All it requires is that you pay attention to your own life; that you realise when you've fallen into one or more of those slow-build habits.

To stop this becoming an ongoing trap, acknowledge what has caused you to get to this point. And don't try to say that you can't help it, or make some other excuse. You *can* help it. Was it not exercising that did it? Too much food? Slow metabolism because you're getting older? Or you simply can't be bothered taking care of yourself? Or perhaps it's a combination of all four. Again, don't try to avoid responsibility. Accept that it's happened – you've put on weight – and resolve to do something about it.

Your next steps are to:

1. Write a food diary (work out how much food you are actually consuming each day).
2. Work out what habits you have (you need to know what you do in order to know what to change).
3. Go through a process of elimination (stop specific habits, if you buy a bottle of soft drink every day after work, buy a bottle of water instead, to keep your energy intake lower then it has been).
4. Work out when you can realistically fit in a bit of exercise into your day, whether it be walking the dog, walk to the post office, riding your push bike for thirty minutes a day or even doing weights at the gym after work instead of heading to the pub.
5. Make small, simple changes in your everyday rituals. Keep them realistic and implement them progressively. I urge you not to go from seven steaks a week with five beers each night to becoming a meditating, yoga-ing vegetarian. That's not a realistic or a sustainable change.

Once you can pinpoint the problem areas and start making progressive changes to your lifestyle and activity level, I guarantee you will see changes in your health.

The upkeep

We've all had those days – maybe for you it's every day: you're flat out at work, leaping from one coffee to the next in need of an adrenaline rush, saying you have no time to eat, yet by 3 p.m. your brain has turned to mush and you can't even remember your own name, let alone the tasks you're yet to complete. Maybe you reach the point where you have the shakes, or start feeling fuzzy in the head and need to sit down, then as soon as you eat you feel ten times better. If that sounds familiar, you've got lots of practice ignoring the red flags your body has been throwing up, all with the same message: FEED ME, FEED ME, FEED ME.

Those shakes, that fuzziness, can often be a result of low blood glucose levels, meaning that there is not enough sugar (otherwise known as glucose) in your system to keep your body energised and your brain functioning at its best. I often see this in people who don't eat breakfast, become busy at work and get their first meal into their belly at 1 p.m. – and by then they are feeling sick.

We all need to keep our bodies fuelled with long-lasting energy foods in order to *have* long-lasting energy. This is where low-glycaemic-index (low GI – you've probably heard of this) foods come in to play.

Energetic eating

It is extremely important to start your day with breakfast. Honestly, I can't believe how often I have to tell people this. You can't start a car when there's no fuel in the tank; you can't catch a fish if you don't bait the hook. So what makes people think they can rocket out into the day when they don't eat breakfast?

One of the best ways to start your day is with a slow sugar-releasing carbohydrate low GI food, such as:

- Raw muesli.
- Bran cereal.
- Wholegrain toast/bread.

All of these foods will help sustain a slow release of sugar into your bloodstream and maintain a normal blood glucose level, giving you energy throughout the morning. Adding protein to this will also provide a very satisfying meal. This can take the form of:

- Raw mixed nuts.
- Yoghurt on your cereal.
- Eggs/cottage cheese on your toast.

The next step is to grab a snack between 10 and 11 a.m., or at least three hours after your breakfast, in order to refuel your system. Try to have a healthy snack, not a donut. Steer away from your vending machine loaded with chocolates, packets of chips and lollies. These types of snacks will not keep you satisfied for long, making you wish for more food or, more likely, more sugar. If you really want a sugary snack, eat some fruit.

By lunch (ideally eaten between 1 and 2 p.m.) you should be jumping back into your lunchbox for:

- Wholesome salad sandwich on grainy bread.
- Bowl of vegetables/salad with some quality protein (see the section on protein that starts on p148).
- A piece of fruit.

By the end of the day you will have eaten five times, getting a snack between each meal, which may prevent you from wanting to overeat when it comes to sitting down for dinner. If you barely eat all day, when it comes to dinner you'll probably eat your entire day's worth of food all at once because you're famished.

If you've established a habit of not eating much during the day you'll have started to progressively slow down your metabolism so, basically, when you're not eating throughout the day, your metabolism almost goes to sleep, saying, 'Wake me when you start to chew'. It does this in the attempt to conserve energy, in case you do not eat again anytime soon – it's an ancient survival mechanism that's still hardwired into our modern bodies. It is believed that your metabolism actually slows down by up to 15 per cent if you have this kind of pattern, and if you also have little muscle, this too will slow your metabolism.

The stored energy or food becomes body fat. I call this type of dieting or starving, 'Camel Syndrome', because, while you're storing water, you *are* storing food. When our body barely eats anything all day and then – wham! – it's given food, it's programmed along the lines of, 'Well, I'd better not burn this off yet, I might just keep this to the side in case I need it, considering I don't eat within ten-hour blocks . . .' And now you have your very own snail's-pace metabolism.

Shift work and food intake

After doing shift work for almost eight years and still occasionally working night duty, I've realised how important it is to be organised when it comes to your food when you're a shift worker.

Try working a twelve-hour day with no food because you forgot to pack your lunchbox, or there was no shop open on the way to work – which can certainly happen when you're going to work in the middle of the night. The next twelve hours can go really slowly, and you end up praying for some spare bread or that half a Monte Carlo will be left in the common staffroom lest you resort to eating your own arm.

Many of the remote workplaces I have visited or had dealings with have no food facilities, except for their beloved vending machines. A few of the men admit that they eat breakfast but don't bother to eat during their shift until they go home, either due to not preparing any food or because they do not feel like eating when they're at work.

The concern I have with this type of habit is that it tends to lead to a desire to grab something quick, which usually means consuming foods high in fat and sugar, or takeaway foods. People who do this tend to run on the highs and lows of blood glucose levels, becoming extremely moody, irritable and fatigued over time. Some people try to power through their shift living on coffee or tea or both – they're really only a quick fix, though, and not at all nourishing. Not only that, you'll often find your sleep during the day is also affected as a result of the amount of caffeine and sugar you've consumed at work.

I highly recommend that when you're on a night shift, eat the same way you do during your day shift. If you eat breakfast, a snack, lunch, another snack and dinner, do the same while on night duties, starting with breakfast when you wake up.

Shift work throws your body out of its cycle, but as long as your body is registering when to eat what meals, you'll keep your energy levels up and your brain power on. Try to stick to quality proteins, vegetables or salads and rice or wholesome grainy carbohydrates in order to keep your blood glucose stable throughout your working day or night. Just make sure your last meal is smaller in size than the earlier meals, because you're likely to be in bed soon after you finish work. And one of the most important things to remember is to consume water. Not soft drink, not 'energy drinks', not beer: *water*.

Try to limit your caffeine intake towards the end of your night duty, although I know 4 a.m. to 6 a.m. can often be the hardest time to stay moving and often this is the time for a quick coffee, but if you can resist you'll feel the difference. You may even sleep better.

Eating out

All of our good food intentions can fall apart when it comes to eating out – particularly eating fast food. Now, I don't endorse fast or junk food but I know full well that you're not going to live the rest of your life without it. Let's be realistic and take a look at the different types of options you have.

> **NUMBER 1 RULE** – Do Not Supersize Anything . . . Coffees, Meals, Soft Drinks, Chips . . .
>
> You don't need it and it is the best way to spend more $$ than intended – it's called clever marketing.

McDonald's – aim for a lean beef burger such as a McFeast. If you head for the salads, forget about the added dressings, or use half the sachet! Spare the fries – do you really need them? If you do – if you really, really NEED them – go for the small option.

Subway® – 6-inch subs should be enough to fill your belly, but whatever size you buy, it's the contents that are important. The healthier option is roasted chicken or roast beef subs, minimising the sauces and melted cheese on top, which instantly increases the amount of energy in the food.

Pizza – no matter which chain you buy from, aim for pizzas like barbecue chicken on a thin crispy base, limiting high fatty-type meats (like meat lovers) with added meats, cheese and bacon. When it comes to eating your pizza, try sitting your pizza on some napkins to mop up any extra oil, plus add a large side salad to the mix. Eating some salad will reduce the amount of pieces you feel you need to eat. Last but not least, do not upsize your meal deal – you'll just eat more than you need.

KFC – something like a chicken fillet burger is actually a better option than the Twisters on the menu. And forget about chips!

Petrol station stops – the next time you fill your car with fuel and you're feeling desperate to fuel yourself too, think wisely about that colourful display in front of you. It's a sure bet that as you pay at the till you're looking at nothing but sugar dressed up in colourful wrappers. Go for the fresh fruit on the top counter, a yoghurt, a high-fibre muesli bar or ready-made sandwich on brown bread with meat and salad. If you have time to sit down and eat, head for the freshly made salad wraps, rolls or a sandwich with lean meat, grilled chicken or steak burgers or even the vegie burgers. The roast dinner is also a better option then many other choices offered in quick stop restaurants.

When it comes to restaurants like Italian and Indian, just keep your choices simple. For entrees, choose options like bruschetta or meat skewers (lamb and chicken). For main courses head for tomato-based sauce pastas or vegetable-based risottos, mussels, roasted and grilled vegetables and meats, choose tandoori chicken or Lamb Rogan Josh. The desserts at the end of the night should be as basic as a coffee and biscotti or a fruit platter or kheer, a type of rice pudding.

At the end of the day, just keep it simple. Trust me, you can't go wrong! . . .

Smart shopping tips

When I give talks and get to the part about the most effective way to shop, I refer to what I call the 'peripheral shop'.

Basically, all the foods your body needs are located in the *peripheral* areas of any supermarket. That means you don't have to dive into the middle aisles for anything – especially Twisties.

Let's start with carbohydrates: as soon as you walk into your local supermarket you come to the bakery section, choosing your bread before entering fruit and vegetable land. Stock up merrily on fruit and vegies, and when making your carb shopping decisions, keep the following in mind.

- Bread – choose wholegrain types, with wholegrain as the first ingredient and more than 3 grams of fibre per serve.
- Cereals – choose wholegrains with at least 4 to 5 grams of fibre and fewer than 10 grams of sugar per serve.
- Crackers – choose wholegrain varieties.
- Pastas and rice – look for brown rice and whole-wheat versions.

Then you walk on to the protein section.

- Beef – choose lean cuts. Aim for labels that say 90 to 95 per cent lean.
- Chicken/turkey – buy skinless breasts/cuts.
- Pork – choose tenderloin or other loin cuts.
- Fresh fish is a great option. In canned fish choose either tuna or salmon in spring water rather than added oils or the new flavours that line the shelves these days (their sodium levels are way too high in comparison to the spring water option).

The only reason for you to walk down the aisles is to buy your pasta and rice, cereals, beans and lentils, tinned salmon or tuna, eggs, toiletries and washing liquids. Some hints for the aisles.

- Canned soups – we all know canned varieties aren't the better option, but hey, I'm trying to be realistic here, especially for you blokes on shift work, or those of you without the ability to cook, remember it's easy, it's quick and much cheaper than your burger option. Choose broth-based soups or chicken/rice and vegetable and choose the low-sodium options.
- Canned Italian tomatoes, tomato paste and tomato sauce.
- Fruit and vegetable juices – 100 per cent juice is best. Select lower sodium vegetable juices.

Try not to buy those pathetic pre-cooked sauces in jars too often – you can make tasty dressings and sauces using olive oil, soy sauce and oyster sauce, along with canned tomatoes. There are less sugars added to these products compared to the 'just-add' sauces which are all too high in wasted kilojoules and way too high in salt (they do nothing to add to the health and energy of your body).

Basic handy hints

- Fresh is best.
- Shop every week (to keep your foods fresh).
- Stock up – the more you have easily accessible, the better. You'll be less inclined to buy takeaway.
- Make your choices colourful – the more colour, the more nutrients.
- Try pre-washed, pre-packed vegetables to make instant meals after a big day.
- Buy walnuts, almonds, sunflower seeds and pepitas for high protein and good fats additional to a meal or snack.
- Use avocado (healthy plant fat) as your new 'spread' instead of using butter or margarine.
- Peanut butter – choose 100 per cent natural options (these are much lower in sodium (salt) compared to the popular brands).
- Dried fruit makes a great snack.
- Frozen fruit like strawberries, raspberries and blueberries also make great snacks

Remember your daily nutrition should be enjoyable – you want to love the lifestyle you lead and the foods you eat. Sometimes you'll have to retrain yourself – you're so used to junk food that you think fresh food doesn't compare. But it's just a matter of training yourself out of it. Yes, junk food tastes good – but, if you *really* think about it, it doesn't taste anywhere as good as a ripe mango or a great piece of barramundi.

The 50 000 km service

Paying attention to what goes into your mouth is vitally important. It's also really important to be familiar with what comes out the other end, because that also tells the story of your nutrition.

When your car goes into the shop, your mechanic (if he or she is any good) will assess the oil from your engine so they can get an idea of the state of the engine and how well it's travelling. When you go to the toilet, the smell and colour of your urine can indicate whether you're getting enough water (hydration) into your system, and your poo (officially known as *stools*) can tell you how well your body is absorbing the foods you're eating. You should know what your regular stools look like – their smell and consistency – and how often you have a bowel motion.

Stools as tools

Assessing your stools can be a great help in assessing your bodily requirements and general health. It is common for blokes to tell me they sit on the toilet for half an hour whenever they need to go – 'and it takes a bit of effort, and my poo looks like rocks, little round, hard things'.

I then ask how much water they drink, and they usually tell me they're lucky to have one glass a day. My initial assumption is that they're dehydrated and the foods they tend to eat do not carry a lot of fluid in them either.

The main role for the small intestine is to absorb nutrients from our foods, and then the large bowel absorbs the majority of the water from foods in order to hydrate our body, leaving what is left: faeces a.k.a. poo.

How often should I do a number two?

People are different, but anything from once every two or three days to three times a day is considered normal. You shouldn't have to strain when you go for a number two. It shouldn't take you any longer than a minute once you have had the urge to go to the toilet in the first place.

From one extreme to the other

There are a number of reasons why you might experience constipation. It does seem to be a little more common in older people but this could be as a result of medications they take, not eating an adequate diet with enough fibre or simply not being able to be as active any more.

For the rest of us, the following may apply:

- Dehydration from not drinking enough fluid.
- Not getting enough fibre into your diet, or even getting too much fibre into your diet but not enough fluid to help the stool travel – this will certainly bulk your stool and make it very hard to naturally travel along the bowel.
- Taking certain medications like iron supplements or pain relievers.
- Being inactive, just sitting around.
- Holding on to a 'motion' because you are unable to go to the toilet for whatever reason (e.g. no toilet available).
- Damage to nerves within the bowel.
- Haemorrhoids or tears which may cause you to want to hold on to a motion.
- Irritable bowel disease, diverticular disease, coeliac disease.

Diarrhoea would be best described as loose bowel motions with urgency – I'm sure you know what I am talking about. There is nothing worse than that panicky need to run to the toilet. If you have ever been to India, you soon get used to people running away mid-sentence with sweat dripping down their forehead . . .

The causes of diarrhoea, besides Delhi Belly, can be:

- Bowel infections.
- Food intolerances or allergies.
- Stomach infections.
- Medications you may be taking to fight bugs.
- Laxatives.
- Irritable bowel disease, Crohns disease, diverticulitis or ulcerative colitis.
- Surgery to the bowel.
- Alcohol.

If you are experiencing any of these symptoms and do not know why, go through this list to eliminate potential causes, otherwise go and see your GP. It's dangerous to let diarrhoea go on for a long period of time because you'll become dehydrated and weak.

Diabetes: the sugar rush that's no fun at all

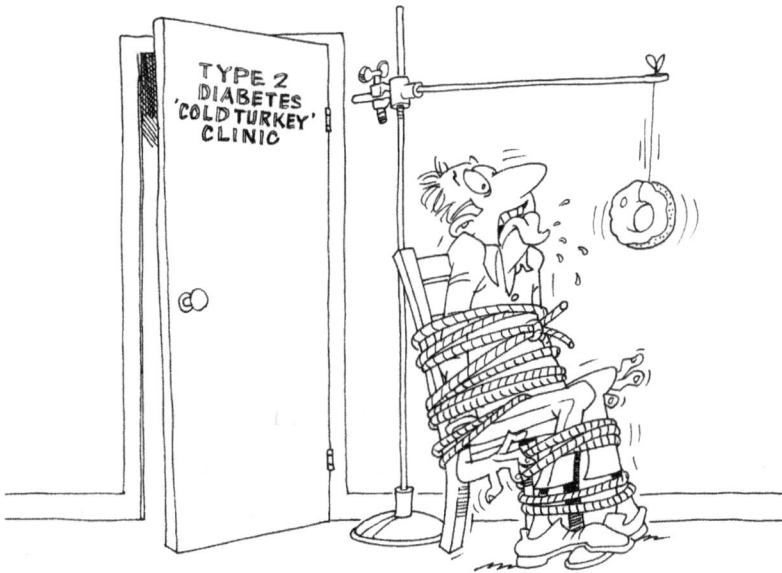

Diabetes is a popular topic in the media – 'fat kids at greater risk of diabetes'; 'too much junk food causes diabetes'; 'sugar addicts at high risk for diabetes'. You tuned out a while ago, didn't you? Not surprising – alarmist articles tend to make people less likely to pay attention, not more. Humans are weird that way.

You probably also tuned out because you think that eating an anti-diabetes diet means you have to miss out on your favourite foods, and that's completely not the case. You just have to avoid becoming a fatty boomba, especially if you become a fatty boomba by eating junk food.

Type 1 diabetics have no choice – they inherit the condition. But type 2 diabetes (which is the type you get from eating badly) is preventable, and there are many good reasons to avoid getting it. Not only will your vision be poor, but if you are not looking after yourself you could end up losing a few toes, possibly even your leg! Are your donuts worth that?

Now that I've tried my own alarmist tactics, let's find out a little bit more about diabetes because even if you don't get it, it's possible that someone in your family will.

The parts

Diabetes happens when your pancreas isn't producing any or insufficient amounts of insulin in the body. Insulin is needed to convert the sugar in the food you eat into the energy needed for your body to maintain its every day functions. In short: no insulin means no energy. No energy means no cricket or footy or shagging or working.

The pancreas

This little organ has the important job of secreting insulin into the blood when you eat food. When you eat, a whole heap of sugar – or glucose – runs into and around our bloodstream. The insulin then zips around the blood vessels to pick up the glucose and converts it into a form of energy.

Let's look at this in a way we can all understand: insulin equals coal.

Let's compare a pancreas to a storage shed, where the pancreas stores all the insulin and the shed stores all the haul trucks (don't tell me that you don't normally park haul trucks in sheds – I'm in charge here).

The sugar (glucose) is similar to coal, giving us our much-wanted energy the way coal powers our electricity supply.

The blood vessels are like the roads within the coal mine. The insulin and the haul trucks need to travel in order to transport glucose or coal around the pit.

The goal for the haul truck is to deliver the coal to specific, designated areas throughout the day. Similarly, as insulin helps to convert glucose into energy, it stores it in three designated areas in the body – our cells, liver and muscles – ready for later use.

As you may know, if coal has already been ripped and pushed by a D11 track dozer, the haul truck still has to transport it back to where it can be converted into energy. This is the same for your body. You can eat all the carbohydrates in the world, supplying the body with sufficient amounts of glucose, but without insulin you won't have enough energy for your body to carry out simple everyday tasks.

When a diabetic eats carbohydrates like bread, pasta, milk and potatoes (these foods supply us with glucose), the glucose that's released into the bloodstream will just sit in the blood until the insulin or insulin-promoting medication is given, allowing the glucose to be converted into energy. Diabetics know to check their blood-glucose level (BGL) throughout the day to ensure they are getting enough insulin compared with the amount of carbohydrates they are eating.

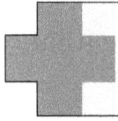

The 50 000 Km service

Some people can be born with diabetes or it can develop later, when they're young children, or even in adult life. They're all different forms of the disease.

The different types of diabetes people can have include:

- Type 1 – better known as insulin-dependent (10 to 15 per cent of all diabetics).
- Type 2, known as adult onset – related to lifestyle choices, but these days we are seeing it in much younger adults, even teenagers (85 to 90 per cent of all diabetics).
- Gestational diabetes, which is caused by pregnancy.
- Pre-diabetes (impaired glucose tolerance).
- Hypoglycaemia (low sugar levels).
- Hyperglycaemia (high sugar levels).
- Ketoacidosis (very high sugar levels, using body fat as energy source).

Now let's break it down. And I'd like you to read all of this because it's highly likely that you or someone you know will have at least one of these conditions at some point. And if it's your child or partner or parent who has it, the more you know about it, the better.

Type 1 diabetes

Most people with type 1 diabetes are most commonly diagnosed during childhood years or under the age of thirty. They are insulin-dependent diabetics who require medication from the point of diagnosis for the rest of their lives, as their form of diabetes is caused by the pancreas not producing enough insulin. Type 1 diabetes is a hereditary condition.

If you're a type 1 diabetic and not taking your insulin (by injection), you're really dancing with the devil. Your body needs energy from somewhere, so if it's unable to get it from the glucose in your blood, it will start accessing energy by burning fat stores. This can be very toxic for the body and can cause your body to go into ketoacidosis, which is extremely dangerous and potentially fatal.

In terms of day-to-day management of the illness, type 1 diabetics generally assess their blood glucose levels (BGL) before they eat. The reading indicates how much insulin they will need at varying times throughout their day or shows that the insulin they are getting is sufficient. They might have to inject themselves with insulin two to four times per day. This is not an injection into the bloodstream – they inject into their skin.

The diabetic's diet and the amount of carbohydrates they eat determine how much insulin they will require. Often people with type 1 diabetes are quite disciplined with their food intake, knowing exactly what they need depending upon the amount of activity they will be doing throughout their day.

How would you know if you have type 1 diabetes?

Type 1 diabetes is usually diagnosed in childhood, so it may be that you're seeing the following symptoms in your child. However, if you're experiencing them yourself you should definitely tell your GP.

- Excessive thirst.
- More frequent urination than normal.

- Constant hunger.
- Blurred vision.
- Unintended weight loss.
- Constant tiredness.
- Skin irritation.
- Cramps.
- Wounds taking a long time to heal.
- Moodiness.
- Headaches.
- Occasional dizziness.

I have met people who, as teenagers, were diagnosed due to constant headaches and vision problems. They assumed they just needed glasses, then their optometrist asked all the right questions and sent them on to their GP, who diagnosed diabetes.

Now what?

If you have type 1 diabetes you need to go from being just a batsman to an all-rounder, because there are a few little jobs you'll have to take on. These include performing prick tests to assess your blood glucose level (BGL) while carefully managing your insulin dosage and daily diet and keeping physically active. Keeping your BGL within the normal range is extremely important for your ongoing health. After a period of time diabetics get pretty good at picking up the warning signs if their BGL is either too high or too low.

The main thing to know is that there's no cure for type 1 diabetes, so you really need to look after your body to prevent any further complications down the track. It doesn't mean you can't drink beer or eat white bread, but you'll have to do everything in moderation. Which isn't such a bad thing, when you think about it. Whatever you do, please don't think you can ignore your disease for one day and have a carbohydrate blow-out or drink two bottles of wine. Because you can't, not unless you want to possibly lose a limb, lose your sight or die. Blunt, I know, but hopefully that's got the message through.

Type 2 diabetes

We used to call type 2 diabetes 'adult onset' diabetes, as the average age of people contracting the disease was between forty and fifty years, who were getting it often as a result of poor lifestyle choices. Now it's starting to show up in young children and adolescents, and again lifestyle choices are to blame.

The difference between type 2 and type 1 diabetes is that in type 2 the pancreas will still secrete insulin, but just not enough or not as effectively as it normally would. This means the type 2 diabetic needs to take medications or insulin to help with the conversion of glucose into energy.

How do you get type 2 diabetes?

Type 2 diabetes is influenced by genetics – if you have a relative with it, you're more at risk than the average punter – but your lifestyle is a huge influence. If two or more of these risk factors apply to you, get thee to a doctor.

- Excess weight.
- High blood pressure.
- If you're over forty-five years of age.
- Not being overly active.
- Eating a consistently poor diet.

- Aboriginal or Torres Strait Islander, Pacific Island, Indian or Chinese background over thirty-five years of age.

If you're carrying a spare tyre around your belly – yes, you, with the four sausages on your plate – you're a good candidate for type 2 diabetes. You really, *really* need to ask yourself whether eating lots of fatty food is worth having a life-threatening condition. Really, really, *really*.

How would you know if you have type 2 diabetes?

The signs are very similar to those of type 1 (see pp183–84).

Often people find out when they go to the doctor complaining about feeling tired or constantly thirsty, or just to have a routine check-up. The doctor may give them a fasting blood glucose test which tells you whether or not you have diabetes.

Now what?

Again, lifestyle plays a big part in keeping this form of diabetes in control, minimising any effects to your body down the track.

If you've been diagnosed with type 2 diabetes you may not need to take medication if you can manage to control your BGL with diet and keeping up with routine daily exercise. And I must add – that modifying your diet and getting some 'huffy-puffy' (as Kath Day-Knight would say) are far preferable to taking medication. Medication may seem like the easy way out, but there ain't no such thing as a free lunch. All medications have side effects – do you really want to *increase* the load on your body? It's easier to cut out your hamburgers and chips. *Yes it is.* Don't give me that.

If you fail to keep the disease under control – if your BGL

never reaches a reasonable level – as you get older and the disease progresses you may then need to take medication. The tablets won't provide insulin; they'll simply help cells utilise the insulin that's already in your body.

If your condition doesn't improve as time goes on – if your pancreas doesn't seem to be delivering enough in order to keep your BGL within the normal range – you may also need to start taking insulin. Don't think you can just start taking the insulin in the kit bag of your mate Bruce from the gym – each person needs individualised medications. You'll need to talk to your GP, specialist or diabetic educator about when you need to take these tablets and/or insulin, and what the regime will be. Make sure you follow their instructions, too. It's not like school. You can't ignore the teacher – not unless you want permanent detention.

Curse my DNA!

If you know that type 2 diabetes is in your family, that's actually good news – you can get the jump on the disease and prevent or considerably delay its onset by living a healthier lifestyle.

At the risk of sounding like a broken record (or a dodgy mp3), you'll need to do the following:

- Regular exercise.
- Maintain a healthy weight.
- Choose the better food options – *yeeeees*, that means things that are green (and I don't mean lime-flavoured milk).
- Manage blood pressure and cholesterol levels.
- Stop smoking (surely you don't need to be told this? Again!).

Pre-diabetes

Pre-diabetes is also another term for 'impaired glucose metabolism'. Pre-diabetes is the name for what happens when the BGLs are a little too high to be normal, yet not high enough to be diabetes. If you're diagnosed with this, take it as a warning – and an opportunity. People with pre-diabetes have ten to twenty times greater risk of developing type 2 diabetes than other folks, but it's not a sure thing. If you take some simple steps to change what you're eating and add some activity to your life, you can steer yourself away from the nastier outcome.

You're more likely to get pre-diabetes if you:
- Have a family history of it.
- Are overweight (carrying visceral fat, known as tummy fat).
- Are inactive.

Are you seeing the pattern developing? Just in case, here it is: DIET AND EXERCISE. DIET AND EXERCISE. DIET AND EXERCISE. These are the two most important things. Now close your eyes and repeat it to yourself three more times.

Hypoglycaemia

You've probably had at least one experience of thinking that you need to eat food NOW NOW NOW or you'll pass out. You'll probably know other people who get a bit that way too. This may be a hypoglycaemic episode, which basically means that your BGLs drop too low, causing you to feel a little shaky or almost faint.

You do not have to be a diabetic to experience a 'hypo'.

Drinking too much alcohol can cause you to have a hypo the next day – ever woken up with the shakes after a night on the tiles, needing food in your belly immediately? But usually it's diabetics who have either had a little too much insulin or not enough food, or who have exercised harder than intended without having the reserves to refuel the body, who are more likely to experience this.

The symptoms

If you're experiencing hypoglycaemia you may be:

- A little shaky.
- Dizzy.
- Sweating.
- Light headed.
- Having a headache.
- Having poor concentration.
- Feeling irritable and frustrated.
- Feeling super-hungry.
- Possibly experiencing numbness.

You may not experience all of these symptoms, but certainly these are the common ones we see on a day-to-day basis when people are experiencing hypos. If it's not you but someone you know who's having a hypo and you know they're a diabetic, don't muck around.

Treating a hypo

Food is generally the best way to treat a hypoglycaemic episode. Go for anything sugary, such as:

- fruit juice;

- jellybeans;
- soft drink;
- honey;
- plain old sugar.

You don't need a lot of these things, according to Diabetes Australia: half a glass of juice or soft drink; or seven jellybeans; three teaspoons of sugar or honey is enough to reverse a low blood glucose reading.

It may take up to 15 minutes before you notice a difference. If there is still no effect, then have another serve of the above foods. Don't give them bread or some other low-GI food – you need a quick-acting sugar that will get into the blood immediately. If you're in a hypo, it's not the time to worry about getting holes in your teeth.

Once the sugar fix has done its job, you can then make sure that there's more sensible, slow-release food, such as:

- a piece of fruit;
- a sandwich;
- a glass of milk;
- biscuits and cheese;
- low-fat yoghurt.

If you know you experience hypoglycaemia often or it has happened a few times, it is important to protect yourself by being prepared. Make sure your family, friends and colleagues know about your situation, so they can be prepared if you suffer from a hypo and need a quick response.

If you're a diabetic or get hypos for some other reason, Diabetes Australia recommends that you carry a 'hypo pack' so you can be treated immediately. The pack should include:

- The name of the person it belongs to.
- A list of the things in the pack.
- A list of hypo symptoms.
- Instructions for how to treat a hypo (for those who may need to use the pack).
- Fast-acting carbohydrate such as jellybeans or honey tubs.
- Slow-acting carbohydrate such as muesli bars, fruit bars and biscuits.
- Doctor and hospital contact numbers.
- Emergency contact details.

If you're with someone who's having a hypo and they're exhibiting slurred speech and poor concentration, call an ambulance. They may become unconscious, and possibly have a fit. Which, as you might imagine, is not so good.

Hyperglycaemia

Hyperglycaemia – a 'hyper' – is caused by high levels of glucose in the blood. It is often the hyper symptoms that make people go to the doctor with questions and soon get tested for diabetes, but often the levels have to be quite high before the symptoms become noticeable.

The symptoms

The symptoms of a hyperglycaemic attack are similar to those of hypoglycaemia (see p189).

A hyperglycaemic episode could occur because you're:

- Stressed.

- Have eaten too many carbohydrates at one time.
- Are ill.
- Have not had the adequate amount of insulin or diabetic tablets.

If you are a diabetic and this is happening to you, visit your doctor to see whether you need your insulin or medications increased.

Ketoacidosis

Ketoacidosis in a diabetic occurs when a diabetic (mostly type 1) does not have enough insulin in their body, and this causes the BGLs to be extremely high. Rather then the body using glucose for energy (as insulin helps the body to convert glucose into energy), the body starts using body fat for energy instead. This might sound a bit handy for various reasons, but having a whole bunch of ketones – which are unleashed when the fat becomes released for energy – floating around in your blood can have dangerous toxic effects on the body.

Ketoacidosis can also occur when a person has an illness or when they're on a strict no-carbs diet.

The symptoms

There are some cheerful little signs that you may have keto-acidosis.

- Rapid breathing.
- Sweet-smelling breath.
- Flushed cheeks.
- Vomiting.

- Dehydration.
- Possible belly pain.

Ketoacidosis is certainly not something you just want to self-diagnose and treat. You need to see your doctor, who will probably test your urine. If you're in ketoacidosis, you're bound to have moderate to high levels of ketones on a 'dipstick' ketone or urinalysis test.

The upkeep

If you're a newly diagnosed diabetic, the question 'What can I eat now?' is probably on the tip of your tongue – if you haven't already grumpily directed it at your doc. The truth is that all of us should eat like diabetics, consuming moderate amounts of good foods. The main thing many diabetics focus on is they can no longer eat their tub of ice cream or sugary sweets, or add their sugars to their coffees. Boo hoo. You already knew you didn't need ice cream to live, and now you're finding out that not only can you live without it, you could die if you continue to eat that tub. You need to deal with it. Once you cut all the sugary stuff out of your diet, you won't miss it – you'll probably even find that your tastes change.

In truth, sugar is not the main focus for restructuring your diet. The big deal is carbohydrates in your daily diet. Carbohydrates are digested and broken down in the body into small molecules of glucose, which our bodies use for energy. So how much carbohydrate you should be eating, the type or quality of the carbohydrate – whether or not it's fruit, bread, rice or lollies – will make a big difference to the amount of glucose released into your bloodstream. The time of day at which you eat these carbohydrates is also important. You want to make sure you start your day with a low GI food, allowing glucose to slowly be absorbed into your bloodstream, giving you a slow release of energy over the course of the morning and again at lunch time and again at your evening meal, not to mention your snacks in between these meals. This will help prevent your 'highs' and 'lows' in glucose world. Check out the 'You are what you eat' chapter for the better food options.

Over the years, diabetics have used the 'carbohydrate exchange' system. They have a certain allowance of carbohydrates within the day, placing foods into 15 g portions of carbohydrates, learning to balance out their carbohydrate load with each meal. As described in the *Diabetes and Pre-Diabetes Handbook* (written by Professor Jennie Brand-Miller, Kaye Foster-Powell, Professor Stephen Colagiuri and Alan Barclay), a 15 g portion of carbohydrate is considered to be a slice of bread, a small piece of fruit and a glass of milk. Now this might sound easy, but this exchanging of carbohydrates can certainly have pitfalls when looking at more complex foods, eating out or using varied recipes.

Carbohydrate counting is another indicator which can get a little complex, yet diabetics seem to do well using this method.

It's not true to say that cutting out carbs altogether solves all your problems with your BGL. Carbohydrates are *extremely* important for your body as they keep you energised and feed the body and the brain – you really do need them. Even if eating carbs means you need to take insulin to help counteract the effect of the carbs in your diet, you are managing to keep a healthy balance in other areas of your health, such as maintaining fibre and essential nutrients for your body.

Why do people talk about a low GI diet and diabetes in the same sentence?

'GI' stands for 'glycaemic index'. Basically this index categorises all carbohydrates into low, moderate or high according to their level of 'digestion and absorption' by the body – that is, how quickly the glucose from the carbohydrate is absorbed into the bloodstream. The rate of absorption determines whether the BGLs rise rapidly or maintain a slow, steady rise.

Any diabetic – and, really, everyone else – should aim for a steady, gentle rise in BGLs throughout the day by eating grain-based breads, complex carbohydrates and fruits, rather than munching on high-spiking sugar hits from foods like chocolate bars or white bread, which cause your BGLs to rise like mountains and then drop like canyons. This kind of white-water sugar ride is what makes people feel tired and irritable, gain weight and continuously feel unsatisfied, looking for more food in the cupboards.

According to the *New Glucose Revolution Guides,* foods within the low GI include raw muesli, porridge, basmati rice, pasta, apples, pears, sweet potato, sweet corn, oranges, noodles, strawberries, peaches, wholegrain/multi-grain breads, nectarines, plums, apricots, rye bread, lentils, red kidney beans, mandarins, sourdough bread, gluten-free muesli and chickpeas. Most vegetables have very little carbohydrate, except for the starch-based options (pumpkins, corn and white potatoes) as already mentioned, so you can chow down on broccoli till the cows come home. Come on, you know you want to.

Foods with moderate GI include angel food cake, risotto, barley, digestive biscuits, shortbread and blueberry muffins.

Foods with a high GI include bagels, white bread, morning coffee biscuits, instant microwave porridge, chocolate bars, lamingtons, desiree potatoes, dates, fruit biscuits and jasmine rice.

If you're a diabetic or you're hoping to prevent yourself getting type 2 diabetes, it's worth adopting low GI eating as a lifelong habit. Low GI foods produce steady results in your weight, helping you lose body fat rather than excess fluid. A low GI diet can also help improve your mental clarity, increase your insulin sensitivity and keep you energised.

Two-thirds of all Australian blokes are overweight or obese. Sixty per cent of diabetes cases could be prevented or delayed by people maintaining a healthy weight. This is fairly simple mathematics. I'm sure you can work out what you need to do.

Gout: is it really God's way of telling me I drink too much beer?

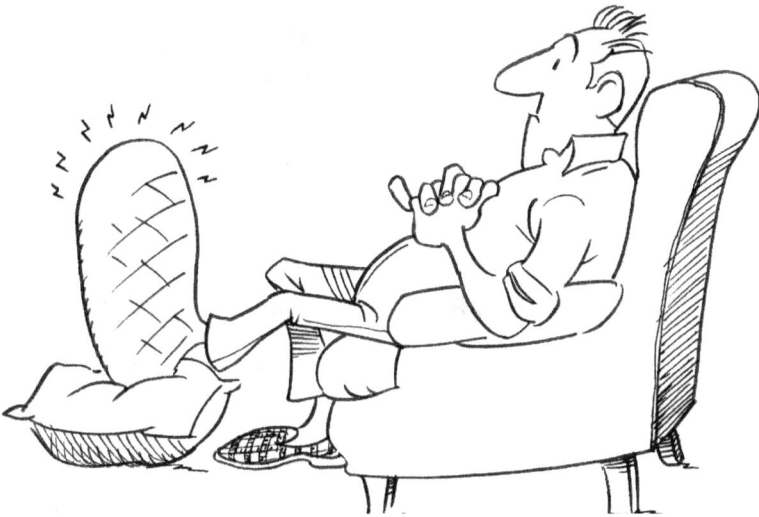

Leonardo da Vinci had it; Leonardo di Caprio may yet develop it. Benjamin Franklin also had it. And you probably know someone who's had it; maybe your own father. Or maybe you're having trouble pulling on your RM Williams boot and wondering why. Well, that reason may be gout.

Gout sounds like something out of Shakespeare's *Twelfth*

Night and that's about right – Sir Toby Belch was the perfect candidate for gout. Gout is one of those wonderful words that let you almost feel the discomfort of the condition just by uttering its name. Go on, say it with me: goooooooouuuuuuuuttttt. Can't you just feel your ankle joint swelling?

The parts

Gout is a common form of arthritis caused by an increased level of uric acid in the blood. The build-up of uric acid crystallises in joints, causing an affected joint to become inflamed, appear red and feel really sensitive (this is a code word for 'painful').

For many blokes, their very first episode of gout will occur in a big toe and if the gout recurs, further episodes will occur in other joints like the ankles, knees and hands. Thankfully, in most cases, gout occurs in one joint at a time.

Who gets gout?

Often gout is considered to be a 'middle-aged rich men's' condition, as you often see it in blokes who enjoy their alcohol and their food. Men who eat a lot of meat are particularly prone, as meat leads to high uric acid levels in the blood, and gout is more likely in blokes aged between forty and fifty. It's also ten times more common in men than in women.

Those most commonly affected are people who:
- Have family members who suffer from gout.
- Are overweight or obese.
- Eat a high-protein diet.
- Have high cholesterol.
- Have high blood pressure.

- Have diabetes.
- Have heart disease.

Some pre-existing conditions can cause high uric acid levels. These include:

- kidney failure;
- psoriasis;
- leukaemia;
- polycythaemia.

Acute attacks can be caused by:

- Alcohol binging.
- Overeating – for example, filling your belly with rich foods on Christmas Day.
- Starvation (I know, it seems paradoxical, but just believe me).
- Surgery.
- Infections.
- Certain medications, such as fluid tablets (Lasix).

The upkeep

Gout lasts for up to seven days, and from the time of onset it tends to improve over the course of the week. In this time you need to see your doctor, drink plenty of water, and avoid foods and alcohol which may be causing further symptoms.

When the acute symptoms occur – joint swelling, redness and pain – see your doctor for medication to minimise the inflammation and reduce the pain. Drink 1 to 1.5 litres of water a day to help flush the uric acid crystals from your body. And there are specific foods to avoid when suffering with gout (see the relevant section on p201).

In cases of chronic gout, a few joints can be affected at the same time. This is known as 'polyarticular' gout and it needs to be treated, otherwise the joints will suffer in the long run. Arthritic joints can really stuff up your golf game – permanently. Best not let it get to that stage.

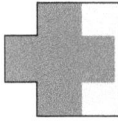

The 50 000 km service

During acute attacks the most effective treatment for gout involves medications for pain relief, inflammation and various types of steroids. Your doctor will advise you on the best medication for your condition.

However, many blokes take long-term preventative treatment to minimise the risk of having further attacks. This treatment includes:

- Medications which help to minimise serum uric acid levels.
- Weight loss for those who are overweight.
- Limiting foods high in purines.
- Reducing the amount of alcohol consumed.
- Drinking more water.
- Stopping medications which may also influence the build-up of uric acid levels.

Ongoing maintenance

It is recommended that people who suffer from gout should minimise their intake of foods containing purines. Purines are considered to be compounds found in certain foods which, when broken down, form waste products – specifically, uric acid.

Foods high in purines include:

- red meat;
- offal (liver, kidney, heart);
- shellfish;
- scallops;
- mussels;
- herring;
- mackerel;
- sardines;
- anchovies;
- yeast-containing foods (such as Vegemite);
- beer;
- drinks containing a type of sugar called fructose (fruit juices or some soft drinks).

It is not proven that by avoiding these purine foods you will avoid attacks of gout, but there can be a connection to eating a lot of these types of foods and an attack occurring. There are some specific fruits and vegetables that appear to be high in purines, but they do not seem to be associated with high levels of uric acid in the body, so we won't put them on the bad list.

Of course, you will probably not want to give up the beers, particularly if you're in the routine of finishing work and having drinks with your workmates or at the golf club, or even beers when you get home. But the bottom line is that beer appears to have high levels of purines, and therefore it's best avoided or kept to a minimum. If you really need to have those drinks, switch to spirits (in moderation, of course). Or, better yet, go on the wagon for a while.

Sex: or, your bits, her bobs and what you need to know about them

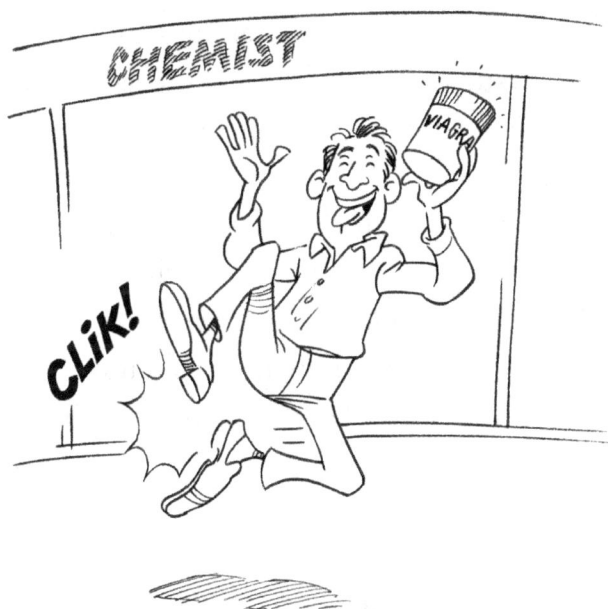

The parts

The early bloomer

What do you mean this isn't your problem? Are you *sure* you've never prematurely ejaculated, not even once? Because one in three blokes – *at least* one in three, given that not everyone will admit to it – has been a little, er, overexcited from time to time. It's nothing to worry about unless it's happening most of the time and, even then, maybe it doesn't worry you. But if it's worrying your missus . . . well, I'd advise you to read on. And read on anyway, because maybe it's your best mate who's suffering in silence. Not sure how you'll broach the topic with him, but you could just hand him this book! Here goes anyway . . .

According to the International Society for Sexual Medicine, premature ejaculation is considered to be 'ejaculation that always or nearly always occurs before or within about one minute of vaginal penetration; and inability to delay ejaculation on all or nearly all vaginal penetration; and negative personal consequences, such as distress, bother, frustration and/or the avoidance of sexual intimacy'. (Palmer and Stuckey, MJA 2008; 188: 662-666)

Put another way: ejaculation is a bit like a car's windscreen wipers. Some work really well while others are a bit hit and miss, working one day and not the next, or simply not working at all. Of course, this really only matters if it's raining. If it isn't raining, it doesn't matter what's going on with the wipers. And, unfortunately, you usually don't know if they're working *until* it's raining. Right?

The problem with faulty *windscreen wipers* – if you get what I mean – is the knock-on effect it can have for both you and your partner. Once it happens the first time, you may feel a slight anxiety about the next time you have sex because you don't want to let your girl, or yourself, down. If it happens a second time you'll have a little more apprehension about a recurrence, or a pattern, and that's when the excuses may start: 'I've had too many beers', 'I've had a big week at work and I'm just too tired', 'I've got stuff on my mind – maybe in the morning, hey'. Does this sound like you? Well, it doesn't have to stay that way.

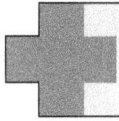

The 50 000 Km service

If you're an early bloomer, first go and see your GP, so long as you feel comfortable with him or her. If you don't, find yourself another one. Then you'll need to actually open your mouth and say what's wrong, and I'm not underestimating how hard that can be. But the doc isn't going to judge you – they will have seen problems a lot bigger (no pun intended) than yours. It's in your interest to be honest about what's going on otherwise they can't help.

The GP will ask you a number of questions before they can diagnose that premature ejaculation (let's call it 'PE' for short) is your problem. Then they can treat you or refer you on to another professional.

Some of those questions may be:

- When did the problem first start and was it associated with any emotion?
- How long (referring to time) into intercourse is it before you ejaculate?
- How many times has this happened or how long has the problem been going on for?
- What were your past sexual relationships?
- How distressed are you and/or your partner about the premature ejaculation?
- Have you had any previous medical problems?

- What, if any, medications you are on?
- Do you suffer from stress, anxiety, depression?

There will also be a physical examination of your bits, and possibly an assessment of your prostate gland (you'll need to just cop that and relax).

Premature ejaculation is categorised as follows:

- Primary premature ejaculation – the problem has been there since your very first sexual encounter and has never changed.
- Secondary premature ejaculation – it has only started after previously having satisfying, problem-free sex.

The causes of PE can vary considerably for each individual. Most commonly there's a mixture of both psychological factors and health problems, otherwise known as biological factors.

The psychological factors may include stress caused by something other than your PE but which means that your mind just isn't on the job; feeling anxious about being able to maintain an erection long enough to pleasure your partner (common in younger, less-experienced males – not you, though, right?); or something else, like feeling a sense of urgency (if you're engaging in al fresco *in flagrante delicto*, say) or simply erectile dysfunction.

Health/biological triggers can include impotence (not being able to get an erection or a lasting erection for a long enough period of time), some medications (ask the doc about this), infections to your urethra (where your urine passes), abnormal hormone levels, inflamed prostate, anatomical discrepancies or even thyroid disorders. Please don't try to take a guess at these yourself. There's someone who spent six years in the prime of their life doing a Bachelor of Medicine who'd really rather you talk to them . . .

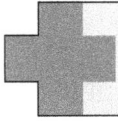

The 150 000 Km service

I'm going to take a wild guess and say that if you're experiencing premature ejaculation, you probably don't want to keep experiencing it (unless it's some kind of fetish, but that's another book). Luckily there are a few options for treatment, from behavioural therapy to counselling, actions to minimise sensation to the penis and pharmaceuticals.

I'm going to start with the one that will probably appeal the least, given that you blokes are mostly allergic to the term 'therapy' – but you shouldn't be, because it's probably more fun than *minimising the sensation to the penis*, eh? So pay attention. Behavioural therapy looks at 'stop–start' techniques, trying to teach you to gain control over your erection and to stop stimulation before ejaculating, allowing the feeling to disappear so you can start the cycle again. Another technique is the 'squeeze technique'. I'm not going to describe that in detail here – I need to leave something for you to ask your GP.

In combination with other treatments, counselling can help you get your head around any self-esteem problems you may be having because of the PE – and it's normal to have valleys and peaks in self-esteem – as well as anything else that may or may not seem to be related to the condition.

Reducing the sensation to the penis is actually not as drastic as it sounds: it can be done by using two condoms at a time during intercourse, so you don't get as aroused. This method will give you a little more control during intercourse. There are also anaesthetic sprays or creams which can be used to numb the head of the penis, which can help to delay ejaculation.

The pharmaceutical options vary but often drugs called Tricyclic antidepressants and Selective Serotonin Reuptake Inhibitors (SSRI) can give a bloke greater control of his sexual pleasure. Your GP is the best person to ask about these because you'll need a prescription.

While you're considering these options, remember to keep talking to your partner. After all, she (or he) cares about you – or, at the very least, cares about their sex life – and they'll want to know what's going on and whether you need some help. Premature ejaculation is never usually a problem if all you're doing is playing solo – it's a team-sport issue.

But wait – there's more!

Premature ejaculation is not the only thing that can make your sex life go haywire. Here are the runners-up.

- Delayed ejaculation – when an extreme amount of arousal is needed to have an orgasm with ejaculation. Yes, mister, this can be classified as a *problem*.
- Anorgasmia – you're unable to achieve an orgasm.
- Retrograde ejaculation – semen actually travels backwards to the bladder rather than out via the urethra. Urine often looks cloudy after sex due to mixing with the semen.
- Anejaculation – no ejaculation at all. Semen is unable to travel from the prostate or seminal ducts into the urethra.

The good news is that you won't get anyone accidentally pregnant.

- Painful ejaculation – pain around the perineum or groin, or in the urethra, during an erection. Often due to a blockage or swelling in the area.

These disorders can be congenital, or caused by abnormal anatomy; psychogenic, infectious or hormonal reasons; as a result of medications, or even social drug use. They are not all that common compared to premature ejaculation, but if you're planning to knock up your wife, they'll need to be attended to. And anorgasmia, in particular, would really suck (this time the pun is intended!).

The crown jewels

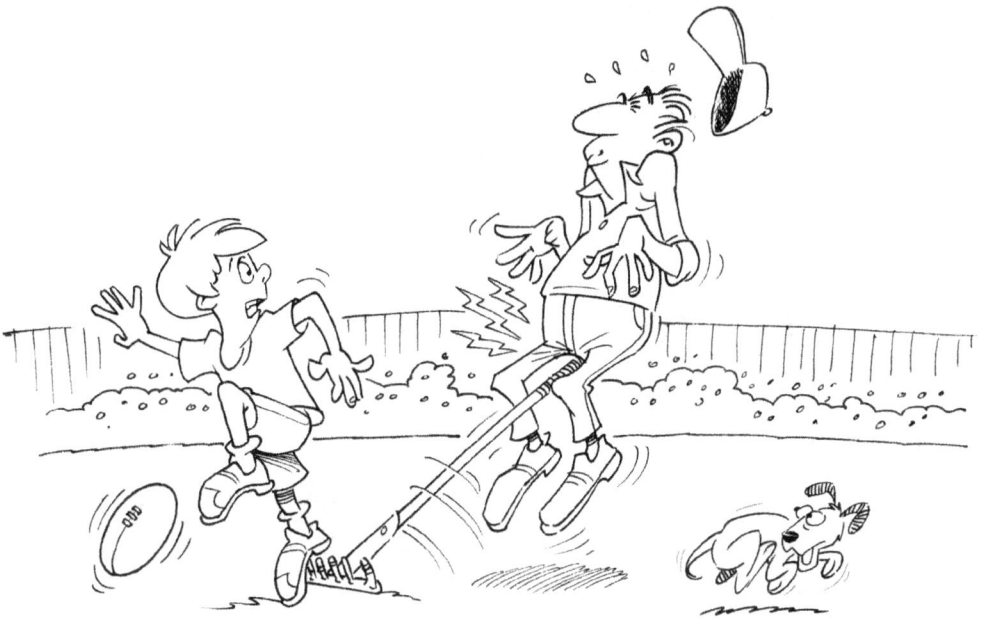

Nuts, balls, boys, 'nads – whatever you call them, every bloke has them (and their proper name is *testes* – or *testi-clays*, if you watch *Little Britain*). And every bloke probably spends one second a day thinking about them – if that – and even then it's probably only when they're getting soaped up in the shower. (Please don't tell me if you don't wash every day!) If you think about them at any other time it's probably in the context of a bit of between-the-sheets fun. Which is a roundabout way of reminding you that your awareness of your crown jewels is not as heightened as they deserve – or need.

The hard fact is that lots of young, fit blokes – and some middle-aged unhealthy ones, too – get testicular cancer. Lance Armstrong is the most famous example, but if you ask around your mates you'll probably find at least one who's had a scare or who has a friend or family member who's lost a nut to the big C. Losing one of your testes is rough, but it's not the end of the world – and it shouldn't mean the end of your life, either, if you read what I'm about to say in the spirit of keeping you from firing on all cylinders throughout your whole life.

The parts

I was tempted to call this section 'Nuts and Bolts' but there's only so many jokes I can make before I wear out my own welcome.

This is the stuff you may already know, but it bears repeating just in case: the testes (meaning the pair), or a testicle (being just one), are small, oval-shaped organs which sit inside the scrotum, the skin sack behind the penis. The scrotum is divided into the left and right sacs.

The testes are in charge of making sex hormones (such as testosterone) and sperm, and the average size of a testicle is 2.5 cm wide and 5 cm long. It's important to remember that the size of the testes – just like the size of your penis – has no bearing on your masculinity or your ability to bear children or to pole vault. The size is coded in your DNA and that's all there is to it.

The tadpole factory

Sperm is made in the testes, so from the testes they swim to the epididymis, which is a long tube – bloody long, actually, at almost 7 metres, which kind of makes this the 1500 m freestyle leg of the journey. From the epididymis the sperm vamoose to the vas deferens, which then propels them into the ejaculatory ducts. These ducts hit the turbo charge to get the sperm into the urethra, where they mix with other fluids from the prostate (that was probably more information than you wanted to know), and then get ready to exit the body . . . and I'm fairly confident you know how they do that.

When the boys go into hiding

No doubt you've had the odd experience of your balls feeling like they've vanished back up into your pelvis – usually when you're really cold or, funnily enough, when you're having an orgasm.

Generally your sperm like to be a little cooler compared to the rest of the body, hence they're stored outside your body. Sperm tend not to tolerate extreme changes in temperature, so when you take a dip in a cold body of water, for example, the two types of muscles in your scrotum contract, causing your scrotum to elevate and retract into the body, helping to keep your sperm warm, comfortable and, most importantly, viable.

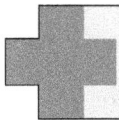

The 50 000 km service

Ever had that feeling like your nuts are all tangled up and it's making you cross-eyed with pain? There's a name for it! No doubt you're delighted to learn that!

Testicular torsion

Testicular torsion (let's call it TT for short) is described as 'sudden and severe pain' in a region where you really don't want there to be even a tingle of unpleasant sensation. If you've never experienced TT, you can probably guess what it feels like – I imagine you won't want to guess for too long. Basically TT is the name for what happens when your testis (generally only ever happens to one at a time) twists from its tube (the spermatic cord), potentially cutting off blood supply to your testis.

Yes, it can happen to you

A TT can happen to any male at any age (babies, infants and teenagers), but is most common in men under 25 years of age. Some guys are more prone then others.

How it happens

A TT can occur when the testicle rotates or twists on the spermatic cord, kind of like a teabag at the end of its string. The twisting results in little blood flow getting to the testis, hence the pain, but if it twists several times, the damage will certainly be more severe.

We don't actually know what the exact triggers are, but some common possibilities may be:

- After an injury to the scrotum.
- After physical activity (not unrelated to the point above – if you play anything in a scrum you'll need to watch out).
- Being out in cold weather.
- During/after sexual activity (sorry).
- During/after sexual arousal (sorry again).

You'll know you have it when . . .

Anyone who's experienced TT will tell you it's extremely painful, to the point you can't deal with it any longer, no matter how brave you are trying to be.

Symptoms include:

- Extreme sudden pain to one testicle that does not go away.
- Pain that can appear to be in the belly (abdomen).
- Swollen scrotum.
- Nausea and vomiting.
- Fever.
- Testis might appear a little higher than usual.

If there was severe testicular pain and it then settled without treatment, it could be due to the testicle twisting and then untwisting itself naturally, otherwise known as 'intermittent torsion'.

Let me say this plainly: there is never a good reason to have sudden and severe pain in your *testi-clays*. So if you do get it, don't ignore it – it's not likely to go away (and if it does, you lose nothing by going to the doc anyway). If you need any motivation to get to the nearest doctor immediately, this should do it. You could lose your 'nad if you don't.

Untangling the jewels

Often a doctor will know you have a TT when they first examine you, although they may run some other tests to rule out an infection. If TT is suspected, the doctor may order an ultrasound or a nuclear scan of the testes. If there is little blood flow visible in the area, this is a good indicator that the problem is testicular torsion. And then, my friend, you're off to hospital.

The only way to fix a TT is to get in there (in the scrotum) to untwist it, and this is a surgical procedure. If the specialist can save the testicle, they may just remove the testes from the scrotum, unravelling the twist in the spermatic cord, placing the testis back into the scrotum and sewing you back up again. The surgeon may sew the outer layer of the testis to the scrotum wall to ensure it will not happen again.

If the testicle has been twisted for too long, it is highly likely it's dead and needs to be removed for your own health, which will mean you have one functioning testicle. It is quite common for a fake (prosthetic) testicle to be put in place for appearance's sake.

Surgery normally takes up to an hour, and you will be told after the surgery to avoid anything too strenuous for one to two weeks and – not the news you'll want to hear – no sexual activity for four to six weeks, although your doctor may have his or her own recommendations.

Don't let the idea of surgery stop you going to the doctor though. Time really is of the essence when it comes to untwisting the tube, as blood supply needs to be returned to the testis as soon as possible. And I'm sure you won't want to put up with the pain for long either.

So why is it such an emergency?

If you can have a testicular torsion treated within a short time after feeling the pain, the doctors can normally save the testicle by returning blood to the organ. But if you leave it past the twelve-hour period without seeing a doctor, the testicle has potentially not received any blood for that period of time and may need to be removed.

Here are some points to motivate you to be a hero, not a zero, and get to the doc quick-smart.

- If the testicle is untwisted within six hours, it can be saved in 90 per cent of cases.
- After twelve hours, chances of saving the testicle fall to about 50 per cent.
- After twenty-four hours, the testicle can be saved only about 10 per cent of the time.

(Source: mayoclinic.com)

In case you weren't fond of maths at school, here's a translation. The longer you wait, the more likely it is that you'll end up with a nickname that includes the words 'one nut'.

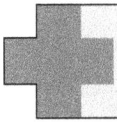

The 150 000 Km service

Unlike other body parts covered in this book, there's not a lot you can do to maintain the health of your testes, other than the general health-and-fitness routine mentioned elsewhere. So I'm going to cut straight to the dramatic stuff: testicular cancer. I hope you're reading this chapter as a cancer-free man and you never need to know what I'm about to tell you. But read it anyway. If you're really pressed for time, read 'The Upkeep' at the end – it's short enough for the ad break.

The basic bits

Here's a few cheerful facts from Cancer Council Australia (2008).

- Testicular cancer is a rare form of cancer.
- It's common among younger men.
- Almost seven in 100 00 men will have testicular cancer.

- Approximately 675 men are diagnosed with testicular cancer each year.
- According to Cancer Council Australia almost half of those diagnosed are under 35 years of age.
- Men aged between 25 and 44 years are most at risk.

And here's the good news. Testicular cancer is possibly one of the better cancers to get – if you can say that about cancer – as it has one of the highest cure rates. If it's caught early enough, you stand a very good chance of complete recovery.

Who's at risk

You have a higher risk of testicular cancer if:

- You have a **family history** of testicular cancer, i.e. if your dad or brother were diagnosed.
- Your **testes** did not drop when you were born or if they still remain **undescended**.
- You have an **identical twin** with testicular cancer.
- You have had an **injury** to the scrotum – although many doctors who diagnose testicular cancer after a trauma believe the tumour may have already been developing but was discovered because of the injury.

It's worth remembering that *no one has no risk* of developing testicular cancer. Don't think you're off the hook – your 'nads are too important to neglect.

The detective work

Quite often when talking to blokes about testicular cancer they've asked me, 'How the hell do you know if you have it?'

Well . . . often you don't. The symptoms can be subtle for some men yet obvious to others. A colleague of mine once told me he found a lump on his scrotum one night when having a shower and had it seen to the very next day. Bingo: it was cancer. As he said, 'I was one of the lucky ones, I acted straightaway, and I was fit, young and healthy'. He did have the advantage of being a medical professional, but you don't need expert knowledge to raise the red flag.

I'm going to tell you some symptoms of testicular cancer, but you're not going to notice most of them unless you're paying attention and giving yourself a regular check. Think of it as giving yourself a good feel in the name of good health.

Symptoms of testicular cancer include:

- An obvious lump in the scrotum.
- A not-so-obvious lump in the scrotum.
- Swollen testicles.
- Aching in the groin.
- Lower backaches or discomfort in your groin or lower belly.
- Your chest or 'man boobs' feeling swollen or painful.

Basically, anything that seems like it's not right is probably not right. And even if it turns out to be something else – like a virus or a sports injury or you're just a bit rundown – it's better not to ignore it. The crown jewels need the royal treatment – you only get the one matching pair and it's easier to hold onto them both if you keep the guards at Westminster. It's better to find out it's just a groin strain, right? Get it checked out just in case. It's possible that your lump is a completely non-threatening, benign little cyst – only a doctor will be able to tell you that. *Don't try to guess.*

Checking your ball bearings

Unlike women, blokes aren't renowned for being highly aware of their lumps and bumps and mole changes – maybe it's because women read more health articles in magazines, or maybe they're just more in tune with their bodies. However, if you're going to learn one self-examination skill I recommend learning to give yourself a good going over downstairs on a regular basis. It doesn't take long, and I'm going to tell you what to look for – just don't take this book into the shower.

First thing to know is that the testes should be almost equal in size. In some men the left testicle might hang a little lower than the right side, and this is nothing to worry about. The testes should feel smooth and kind of rubbery, and they're shaped a little like a boiled egg. As the Cancer Council Australia suggests, from puberty men should be aware of how 'lumpy' their testicles are, in order to note any changes that may occur later in life.

Now to the assessment part. Be gentle with your jewels, and take each testis with both your hands. Use your thumb to glide over the top of the testes with your fingers supporting underneath the testes while you gently roll them and feel for any tiny lumps.

You also need to check out your epididymis, which looks almost like a seam running from the top of your testicle to the back.

Remember that the lumps you want to know about can be the size of a pea, and they're not necessarily painful either. They could be on the side or the front of the testes.

Of course, there is another way to check out your 'nads: have someone do it for you – and I don't mean a doctor. Yes, lads, if you have someone in your life who visits that part of your body more than you do, they are bound to notice changes. Body assessments might become a little more appealing and less of a chore!

If your doc asks what's up

If you have some symptoms and you've done the smart thing and gone to your doctor, he or she will carry out a physical examination of your scrotum and they may then wish to refer you to a specialist – a urologist.

The urologist may want to do some tests: an ultrasound, some blood tests to find any specific 'markers' and, depending on these results, they may wish to book you in for a biopsy to confirm their findings.

If the ultrasound shows a lump, the urologist may take a biopsy from the lump or if it appears to be a cyst, they will drain the fluid from the cyst. If the lump is highly suspicious the specialist will want to surgically remove the affected testis as soon as possible in surgery to examine the type of cancer, in order to eliminate the risk of the cancer spreading to other areas of the body.

To rule out that the cancer has spread, the specialist will request you have what we call a CT (computerised tomography) or MRI (magnetic resonance imaging) scan in order to check out the rest of your body. Both these tests simply require you to lie still on a bed while the machine takes pictures of you.

You may not have everything in common with Lance

You'll probably only be reading this bit if you or someone you know has already been diagnosed with testicular cancer. It's not a comprehensive guide to the different cancers – it's just a heads-up that there's more than one type. But they ALL need to be treated.

The types of testicular cancer differ according to where the cancer cells started in the first place.

The most common, found in up to 90 per cent of cases, are the germ cell carcinomas, otherwise known as non-seminoma or the seminoma carcinomas ('carcinoma' is another word for cancer).

1. Non-seminoma: considered to be a little more aggressive then the seminoma cell carcinoma and often seen in younger men, those in their teens to twenties.
2. Seminoma: considered a slow grower, it is rare for it to spread to other parts of the body.

The other less common type of testicular cancer is caused by stromal tumours, known as leydig cell tumours and sertoli cell tumours. These types of tumours rarely spread, but if they do they are often hard to treat.

So I'll say it again: EARLY DETECTION SAVES LIVES, PEOPLE!

Joining Lance's club

If you've had all the tests and the diagnosis isn't great, the good news is that a swift, effective treatment is available. Unfortunately, it's not one you're necessarily going to like: it's the removal of the affected testicle, otherwise known as an orchiectomy or orchidectomy. And if the cancer hasn't spread, this might be the only form of treatment you will need. Of course, it does leave you a little bit . . . lopsided. This may not bother you, and you probably won't know if it'll bother you until you're actually in the situation. But if it does, ask your doctor about having a prosthetic testicle inserted to replace the original testicle and balance out the scrotum.

I'm guessing, however, that how your scrotum looks is probably not going to be the first thing on your mind. No: if you're a young bloke looking to breed one day, you're probably wondering whether having a testicle removed is going to damage your baby-making abilities. The short answer is 'No'. So long as you have the other testicle remaining, you'll continue to produce sperm. You also won't have any problems with erectile function . . . I've included that in the prostate chapter.

If you lose both testicles, though, you will lose your ability to make sperm. You'll need to talk to your friendly urologist about your options. Sperm can be harvested and stored for possible future use with a partner, otherwise known as pre-treatment sperm cryostorage.

Apart from surgery, other treatments include radiotherapy, chemotherapy, drug therapy and possibly more surgery.

Radiotherapy is no picnic but it *is* effective for killing cancer cells in specific areas of the body. It is a quick procedure, often targeting affected lymph nodes to prevent further spread, and it's effective for those with seminoma cancer cells.

The chemotherapy is often used after radiotherapy, generally if the cancer has already spread or if the testicular cancer comes back. There's no way of making chemo sound good: it's a dirty business. But it can be extremely effective, even if you end up with a number zero haircut for a while.

If the urologist requests further surgery, this may be due to the cancer affecting lymph nodes at the back of the abdomen. So the aim is to get rid of these lymph nodes to limit any further damage or any further spread of cancer cells.

Please bear in mind that none of this may happen to you – if you have a lump, it may turn out to be nothing. If you think not telling your doctor means you will avoid chemo, think again. You may lose a nut but it's better than losing your life.

The upkeep

One last time, here's what you should be doing. SO DO IT. It takes less time than taking a sip of beer.

- Check yourself regularly. Make it a routine – like the first Monday of every month – or ask your lover to check you instead.
- Know your 'lumps' in your testis so you can then detect any changes over time.
- It's best to do the check after a warm shower or bath, when the scrotum is relaxed.
- Know whether you're at higher risk than other blokes (see 'Who's at risk' on p218).

Most importantly: if you find a lump, *don't panic and don't ignore it*. It's probably nothing, but it's better to know that for sure – don't add stress to your life unnecessarily, and worrying about a lump is certainly stressful.

Secret women's business

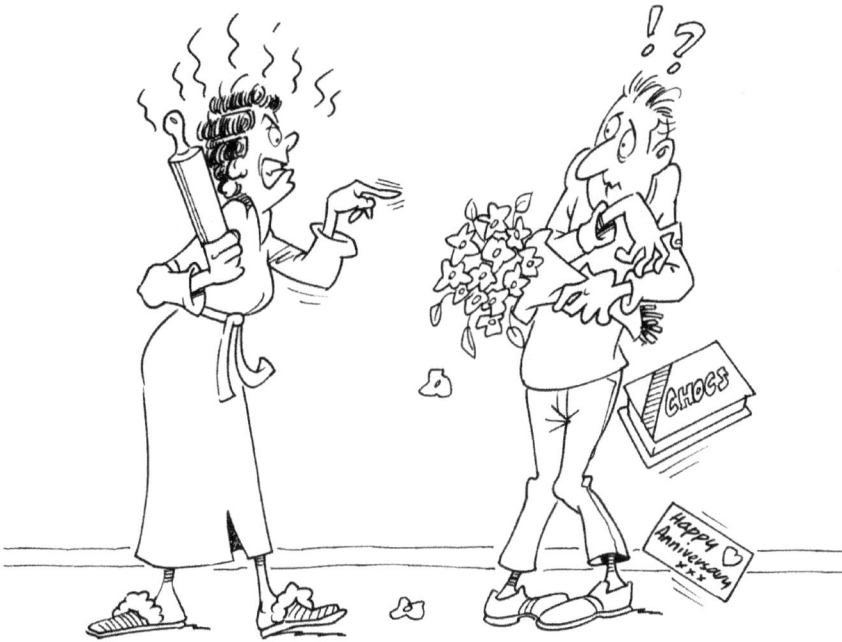

This chapter is about women's business. Even if you're gay, there will be a woman in your life – your mum. And possibly a sister or two, and a good female friend. If you're straight, you may well be married to or shacked up with a woman who has borne you children, and you may be the father of a daughter. So you need to know something about the reason why women's bodies throw up more challenges than men's, and how you can help the woman or women in your life navigate them – and the more you can support them, the sweeter life is. Ever heard the phrase 'Happy wife, happy life'?

The parts

I'm sure you're comfortable with your own tackle but it's well known that even devotedly heterosexual men can lose their way in the map of Tassie, much to the disappointment of the woman it belongs to . . .

It's time for a little anatomy lesson. Yes, yes, you probably heard it all in Year seven biology. That was a while ago – time for a refresher course. Stay with me – it'll be fun! The more you know, the more likely you are to impress.

1. Ovaries

- Similar to two little baskets, one on either side of the uterus in the pelvis.
- Tiny, on average 3.5 cm in length to 2 cm in breadth.
- They are sex glands which produce eggs and hormones (oestrogen, progesterone and androgens). They're busy a lot of the time.
- They're the female version of testes. In fact, your testes started as ovaries when you were still a foetus.
- The ovaries grow through puberty to reach their standard size and start to shrink with age.
- Their main job is to produce an egg each month for potential fertilisation. If not fertilised, the egg will shed via a menstrual period a.k.a. 'having the painters in'.

2. Fallopian tubes
- Hollow tubes allowing the egg to travel from the ovary to the uterus.
- There is one for each ovary.
- They are 10 cm long from the uterus to the ovary.
- There are tiny finger-like projections at the ends closest to the ovary.
- Fertilisation of egg and sperm happens here.
- The tube slowly propels the fertilised/non-fertilised egg towards the uterus.
  Have you ever heard of an ectopic pregnancy? This is often due to the fertilised egg implanting itself halfway along the Fallopian tube before arriving at the uterus.

3. Uterus
- Also known as the womb, usually in the Bible.
- It's pear shaped, 9 cm in length to 6 cm wide. During pregnancy its muscle will stretch to an impressive 40 cm in length.
- It's lined with endometrium (a type of tissue with lots of blood supply).
- A fertilised egg will implant into the wall of the uterus, allowing the development of the foetus.

4. Cervix
- The narrow entrance leading toward the uterus.

5. Vagina
- The opening of the female genitalia leading towards the uterus, located directly below the urethra (the exit path for urine).
- It's 9 cm long.
- If a woman is menstruating this is the exit path for the

menstrual fluid; it's also, unsurprisingly, how babies exit the uterus and enter the world. And you'll know this one: it's where the penis goes during sexual intercourse.

Getting the painters in

Young women usually get their first menstrual period between the ages of 11 to 14. From that age until menopause – in their late forties or early fifties – they'll have a period anywhere from every three weeks to every two months (the average is every 28 days) unless they're pregnant. Let's face the facts, fellas, an average woman can spend almost ten years of her life having her periods . . . no wonder they can have the occasional bad day.

No woman enjoys getting her period, which is something that not many blokes ever consider. A period can last for three days or seven and sometimes doesn't happen at all if the woman is pregnant, highly stressed or has been exercising excessively or not eating properly. It's something every woman just 'puts up with' and there can be all sorts of complications that go along with them which means that the woman or women you know may have a hard time of it. It's worth you taking a few minutes to find out why.

The menstrual cycle has an official start point at day one – the first day of the period. When one period is finishing, specific glands in the brain send hormones preparing the ovary to stimulate the growth of little egg follicles. It may take up to fourteen days for the egg follicles to grow, ready for the next stage. In this time the lining of the uterus becomes nice and thick – preparing itself in case the egg has a chance to be fertilised.

There is (usually) only one egg follicle – the largest-growing follicle – which is forced out into the Fallopian tube in quite an explosive fashion, in order to travel towards the uterus. This is called ovulation.

Some of you will come to know ovulation intimately if you're 'trying' for a baby. Some women – and, by extension, their babydaddies – who are 'trying' for a baby know the hour, or the minute, when ovulation occurs. One clear sign is that the woman will normally experience a higher-than-average body temperature at this point of her cycle.

If the egg isn't fertilised the remaining follicle and its little follicle buddies that lost the race die, causing the levels of oestrogen and progesterone – produced during and following ovulation – to fall. Once this starts to occur, the uterus lining (the endometrium) will shrink over the following seven to ten days.

Now this is what I find the most interesting part: the vessels supplying the uterus with its blood flow also shrink and start to break away, causing small amounts of inconsistent bleeding which warn the woman that her period is soon to start. At this point the endometrium starts to separate from the uterine wall, shedding into the uterine cavity, ready to exit through the vagina once the uterus contracts. It is now time for what is so imaginatively called 'the period', a.k.a. 'rags', 'monthlies' or 'the curse'.

Under the bonnet

Knowing what is happening with the internal mechanics of a woman may help you understand why some women can experience severe cramps or be unable to sleep during this time of their cycle. For some women, their period is painful and distressing.

The term 'premenstrual syndrome' (PMS) – which I am sure many of you have heard – describes the handful of days before their period starts when the women in your lives are experiencing severe hormone level imbalances, pain or emotional swings, from sad to angry and frustrated. It often starts after ovulation, when the endometrium starts to shed, and can last throughout the period itself. PMS can be a real problem for many women; most women have some form of it and even if it's mild it can make life difficult for a while.

The extent of the severity of PMS can be affected by stress and diet, so that sometimes you'll find your normally calm and steady wife or daughter or sister is sad and cross for several days. Instead of taking it personally, try to understand that she's experiencing body changes that may be a little too overwhelming for her; she may be barely coping with her own company, let alone anyone else's. The menstrual cycle can often feel like a curse to many women, and the knowledge that they have to put up with it for forty years or so doesn't help.

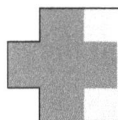

The 150 000 km service

I was once told by an attendee at one of my talks – let's call him Greg – that he felt like he was married to a stranger for almost twelve months, and this scared him . . . and his wife. Neither of them knew what was going on. He explained that he would leave the house for work in the mornings with a kiss from his wife and arrive home having to duck for cover from a completely different woman who looked exactly the same.

Greg admitted to thinking at one stage that he might just have to leave his wife, as he didn't understand what was happening to their relationship. Finally he asked her, 'What is it I am doing to make you so angry and upset lately?' His wife broke down and told him, 'I don't know what is wrong with me. I feel like another person.'

They both decided to go and visit their local GP to ask what could possibly be happening, and whether his wife was sick. The GP asked questions about Greg's wife's moods, energy levels and when she felt the changes had started. Then he asked about her periods . . . BINGO!

The GP announced, 'You're going through menopause.' Greg told me that he and his wife were so grateful they could finally pinpoint the cause, as they had honestly started to believe that she might have had a brain tumour. After attending my menopause talk in his workplace he pulled me aside to say, 'If this can get through to a few of these blokes it may just save a few marriages. I didn't know anything about what to expect, what my wife was going through and she didn't even know what was going on . . . It's real life . . . for all of us.'

Now, your missus may have just had baby number one and be decades off menopause, but what about your mum? She's either been through it or about to go through it. And if you're married to a woman around the age of fifty, you really need to read this next bit. And . . . even if you think you'll never need to know this information, read it anyway, because only monks spend their lives completely without women at home or in the workplace. Once you know a bit more about the things women have to put up with just to ensure the survival of the human race, you may be less hasty to call one of them a 'cranky bitch'.

Here are a few important definitions to help you understand more about menopause. Stop yawning!

Peri-menopause – this is 'around the time of menopause'. The woman may have inconsistent periods over a gradual period of time, with three or four months of no period and then suddenly the painters are laying down ground sheets. It is very different for each woman and can begin ten years before the official last period.

Menopause – this is the term given when there has been an absence of menstrual periods for twelve consecutive months.

Post-menopause – this is the time after the last menstrual period. Women may refer to themselves as post-menopausal – well, they are post-menopausal for the rest of their lives once they have endured menopause.

Just to make sure you're getting this, the next section is going to be in a Q&A format for easy reference. Here we go . . .

1. Why do women go through menopause? (And no fellas, it is not because they deserve it.)

Menopause is the result of ovaries no longer functioning as they once did. One of the ovaries' main jobs is to produce hormones; as a woman ages the ovary shrinks, producing smaller amounts of two important hormones, oestrogen and progesterone.

2. Are these hormones (oestrogen and progesterone) important?

I'm flabbergasted that you need to ask, but since you did . . . yes, fellas, you should appreciate them. It is these two hormones that help make women look different to men. They develop such feminine characteristics as:

- Breasts.
- The shape of a woman's body.
- Body hair (obviously in all the right places i.e. not on their backs).
- Regulation of the menstrual cycle.
- Creating the ideal environment for a pregnancy.
- And did I mention breasts?
- Oestrogen is also very important for the protection of the bones.

3. What age are women when they go through menopause?
This depends on the individual. For many, it is between the ages of forty-five to fifty-five, but for some, menopause may occur as early as their thirties or as late as their sixties. According to various studies, often the best indicator of when a woman will go through menopause is her mother's age at menopause. It is likely that the daughter will experience menopause not at the exact age but around a similar time.

4. What are the symptoms of menopause?
It can vary for so many women, from mood changes to hot flushes as well as vaginal and urinary symptoms.

Hot flushes tend to get the most bad press – and no, I'm not talking about her heating up at the sign of your half-naked body in dirty footy shorts and old socks. Usually the flushes are floods of perspiration, to the point where they – and I quote – 'need a mop', lasting for 30 seconds to a few minutes. They normally happen around the face and neck, or sometimes on the entire body, and can occur during sleep, requiring a towel to be placed underneath the woman in order to soak up the excess sweat. But not only is the excessive sweat, with little warning, hard to deal with for a few of these women, the embarrassment that goes along with it can be quite distressing for many. As one woman told me, 'Flushes give no warning, they do not discriminate, and they tend to like to appear at the most inconvenient times'.

Other symptoms of menopause are so varied that it can be difficult for a medical practitioner to prepare a woman for what they are going to experience. However, the most common seem to be hot flushes, night sweats, overheating, vaginal dryness, skin dryness, irritability, low energy levels, depressed mood, anxiety, low libido, weight gain, poor memory, breath odour, osteoporosis, tinnitus, crashing fatigue, incontinence, aching joints and/or muscles, increased tension in muscles, breast tenderness, headache change, tummy upsets, hair loss/ thinning, increased facial hair, dizziness, body odour, electric shock sensation, tingling in limbs, bleeding gums and burning tongue.

Bet you're glad you're a man. And try to be a bit sympathetic if your menopausal wife, mother or sister has even one of these symptoms. It's not something they're *choosing* to go through.

5. Will menopause affect our sex life?

Yes.

Oh, you want details?

Menopause can affect a woman's sex drive, but it really does vary among individual women. As I have said to people in my classes, 'It is about communication with your partner, learning your partner's body all over again, what works and what doesn't'. However, in order to make this work, both of you need to be

talking about your experiences honestly and openly. If your wife/
partner doesn't think she can trust you, she's more likely to just
stop having sex altogether rather than trying to negotiate the
change. Which scenario would you prefer? Yup. Think of it as a
chance to learn some variations on your old themes.

Due to lowered levels of oestrogen being released in the body
during menopause, there are changes to a woman's physicality
and emotions which can adversely affect her sex life. For
example, she:

- May not be as easily aroused as she once was.
- May be less sensitive to touching and stroking.
- Will have lowered blood supply to the vagina.
- Will not have adequate vaginal lubrication.

Any one of these – and particularly the last item – can make
sexual intercourse very painful. Either learn to make friends
with lubricant or accept the fact that your techniques south of
the border have to change, or both.

Other factors that may cause decreased libido include:

- Bladder control problems.
- Sleep disturbances.
- Depression or anxiety.
- Stress.
- Medications.
- Health concerns.

It's worth remembering that once she's post-menopausal her
experience of and attitude towards sex may improve. But menopause can last for months and years, so if you want some nooky
in the meantime, get creative and learn to listen to what she's

telling you. Remember that it's *in your interest* – you get action if you put in just a little bit more effort. Small price to pay, really.

6. Isn't there a pill she can take?

Kind of. There isn't a pill that can make menopause go away, but there are treatments that can alleviate the symptoms women experience. These include:

- Hormone replacement therapy (HRT).
- Oestrogen and progesterone therapy.
- Oral contraceptive pills.
- Antidepressant medications.
- Alternative therapies (e.g. acupuncture).
- Vitamin E.
- Herbal remedies.

There are also plenty of lifestyle factors that can help control the symptoms and complications of menopause. Some of them would be good for you too, such as getting lots of regular exercise, which is vital for lifting mood and feeling a little more energised, along with eating a healthy, well balanced diet – so lots of fresh fruit and vegetables and great sources of lean protein as recommended by the Australian Guidelines for Healthy Eating.

It is important for your wife, partner, sister or close friend who might be experiencing a difficult time with their menopause to see their GP or health professional, as he or she can guide them to the better options most suitable to them.

It's also crucial for you to be kind and understanding to the woman in your life at such a time. Yes, she may be moody and occasionally out of control. She may not feel like doing some of the things she loves – including getting between the sheets with you – but don't take it personally, because *it's not about you.* It's about her. It'll be over soon enough, and in the meantime if you send a kind word or a soft gesture her way, it'll make the world of difference as to how she feels – and the sort of experience you'll both have. And that's the part that IS about you. Who knows, maybe if you make the effort you could be pleasantly surprised and well rewarded.

The curse of the sun

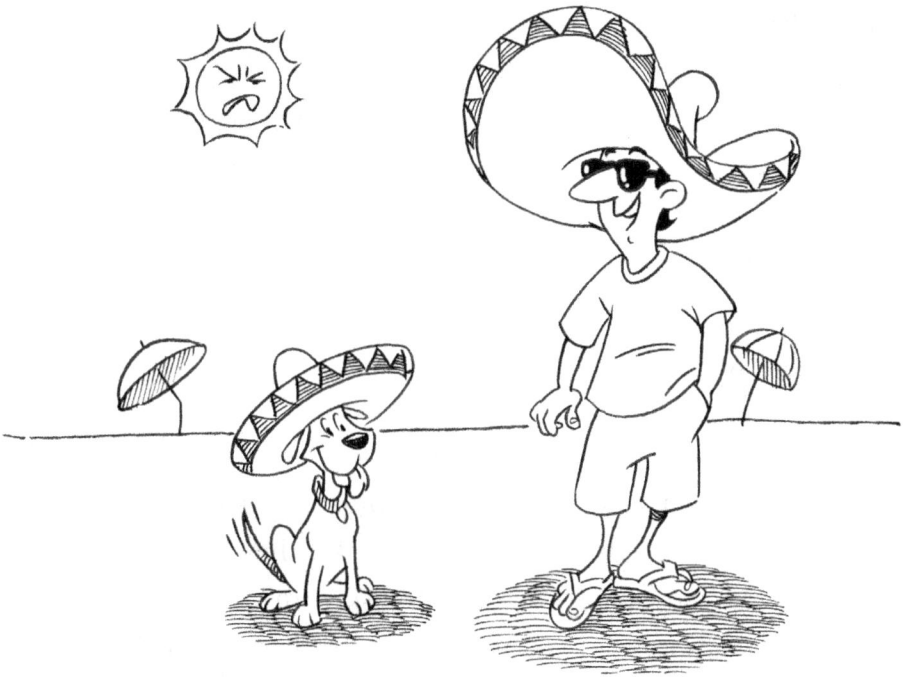

There are many benefits that come from living in this wide, brown land with its pitiless blue skies, far horizons and jewel-like sea. Skin cancer is not one of them. Caucasian skin – or any skin tone that isn't dark – doesn't really belong under the harsh southern sun. Living in this country, we have to keep an eye on our skin and take some precautions to prevent skin cancers, a.k.a. The Aussie Curse.

Skin cancer rates in Australia are the highest in the world. The Commonwealth, State and Territory governments spent $294 million in 2001 promoting skin cancer awareness and research, yet still the rates climb. Maybe our casual lifestyles and the fact that we have mostly fine weather (although that's changing) are to blame – we want to make the most of the outdoor life, even if it's causing greater harm to our health than what we had ever intended. None of us wants to give up our afternoon barbecues, our days at the cricket or lazing about on the beach – we don't have to. We just need to be smart about it. *You* need to be smart about it.

Maybe we just don't understand enough about skin cancer to appreciate that we need to take care. So here goes . . .

Your skin

The skin is the largest organ of our body – it has the greatest amount of surface area of any other organ . . . It's quite similar to the paint on your car. If the sun can lift the paint from your panels, imagine what it can do to the skin on your arms.

If you really care for your car you probably polish it regularly, with the aim of preventing damage to the paintwork which may cause it to become dull or to stop it developing rust. Skin cancer is like rust. If you treat your car so kindly as to buy it a Car Bra, protecting it from surface chips and scratches, stopping it from looking older then it actually is, what are you prepared to do for your skin? All you really *need* to do is wear a shirt and a hat, and use some sunscreen. And I'm sure you only use good quality polish on your car on a regular basis, for maximum effect and protection, so take the same approach to your sunscreen. Please remember that coconut tanning oil is *not* sunscreen. You wouldn't pour oil on your car and then leave it out in the sun, so don't do it to your body.

Skin cancer

Skin cancer is simply a disease of the body's skin cells, resulting from continued exposure to the UV rays from the sun, otherwise known as ultraviolet radiation (UVR).

The top layer of skin is called the epidermis and underneath that is the dermis.

Each layer is made up of different types of cells, with varying roles to play, all of which are important.

The dermis is responsible for our hair follicles, sweat and oil glands, blood vessels, our nerves and lymph vessels.

The epidermis is made up of three types of cells: basal cell, squamous cell and the melanocytes. These cells act as a barrier to the rest of our body, protecting our skin from the heat, the cold and the chemicals in our environment. The type of cancer you may have depends on which cells have been affected

Melanin, produced by the melanocytes, gives our skin its colour, causing pigmentation; every time we are in the sun the melanocytes will produce more melanin, causing the tanning effect which gradually darkens the skin, absorbing UVR.

When skin cancer develops it usually affects one of the cell types within the epidermis, causing cells to multiply abnormally, forming a malignant tumour. The three common types of skin cancers include:

- basal cell carcinoma;

- squamous cell carcinoma;
- melanoma.

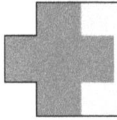

The 50 000 km service

According to Cancer Council Australia, basal cell carcinoma (BCC) and squamous cell carcinoma (SCC) – otherwise referred to as non-melanoma skin cancer – are the most common of the skin cancers and appear to be the least aggressive. Melanoma is the least common yet the most dangerous, in terms of its ability to rapidly grow and spread throughout the body.

Basal cell carcinoma

Basal cell carcinoma is slow growing and painless. It is most typically found on the face, neck, back and shoulders, and the back of your hands. If you have a BCC you may think it is an ongoing ulcer with a shiny, raised surface.

You're more likely to have BCC if you're over forty, unless you're out in the sun a lot – if you're a surfer or a builder, for example. The best form of treatment is cryotherapy, which freezes off the cancer with liquid nitrogen. It's a quick and simple procedure.

Here's a simple tip to prevent BCC developing on the back of your hands: apply sunscreen on your hands when you're driving. You'd be amazed how exposed your hands are, even on short trips. This one simple act could save you a whole lot of freezing!

Squamous cell carcinoma

These little buggers are responsible for 20 per cent of the skin cancers diagnosed. They're rough but slightly tender to touch, slow-ish growing but faster than BCCs. They appear reddish to brownish in colour, can sometimes be ulcerated and may easily bleed if you pick at them. They're commonly found on the lips and the ears, and they need to be treated immediately.

You're at greater risk of getting SCC if you're in the sun regularly over long periods for many years so, often, the older you are, the greater the risk. You need to be particularly careful if you work on the land, if you're an outdoor council worker, truck driver . . . you get the idea.

You can also be at greater risk if you have a poor immune system – for example, if you have an illness which causes immunodeficiency. These illnesses include AIDS, lupus, Sjogren's syndrome and hepatitis C.

Treatment for SCC is certainly possible; the treatment options vary according to the size of the SCC, the location and how long it has been untreated.

Malignant melanoma

Melanoma is the least common type of skin cancer, with less than 5 per cent of total skin cancer diagnoses, but it's the most aggressive – it's responsible for 80 per cent of skin cancer deaths. Around 9500 Aussies are diagnosed with melanoma each year, and more than 1100 die of melanoma each year. Melanoma is the fourth most common cancer in males; there were 2024 Aussie blokes diagnosed with melanoma in New South Wales in 2005, and the survival rate for males diagnosed with melanoma after five years was 89 per cent.

Melanoma may appear in an existing mole or freckle. It may feel a little itchy and bleed, the diameter is normally greater than 6 mm, with noticeable changes to the edges of it, and has definite colour changes over a matter of months.

One in twenty-four blokes will develop melanoma by the age of seventy-five. That doesn't mean you shouldn't think about it if you're under seventy-five – you need to be sun smart *now*. People at risk of melanoma can be young, old, those with fair skin, those with dark skin, those with lots of freckles or moles, and those who get sunburn without even trying.

The best treatment option is for the melanoma to be removed altogether, as these suckers tend to grow extremely quickly, and need to be identified and treated in the early stages to prevent further problems – if a melanoma isn't detected, it will grow rapidly throughout the body.

You may not realise that melanomas aren't only located on areas exposed to the sun – they are generally located on either the legs of women or the upper body on a man. Basically, though, they can appear anywhere.

Your DNA and other cancer-causing agents

You'll have a greater risk of developing skin cancer if you:

- Are out in the sun a lot, either due to work or pleasure.
- Do not cover up from the sun.
- Have a family history.
- Have lots of moles on your body.
- Are an Aussie kid who grew up running around uncovered in the sun.
- Have fair skin with freckles and you burn easily.

- May not see the sun often, but when you do you're happy to burn.
- Have had sunburn.
- Were sunburnt as a child, either frequently or infrequently.
- Have red or fair hair, or blue or green eyes.
- Have sun spots.
- Have weakened immune system as a result of illness.

People with dark skin are still at risk of skin cancer although, due to their higher levels of melanin, they do tend to have more protection than the average fair-skinned person.

Self-service

The 'take-home message' – as some marketing types like to phrase it – is that you need to check your skin routinely and have it checked by a professional every year.

To check your own skin, you first need to *know* your skin so you can notice any changes that may occur over time. The Cancer Council Australia recommends you check your skin every three months, from top to bottom, even looking at the soles of your feet and under your nails. Ask your missus or somebody else to check through your scalp – then you can do the same for them – and use a mirror to see those hidden areas. If it all sounds a bit like chimpanzees grooming each other, you're not far off – after all, they're our relatives so no surprises there.

Ideally you want to be looking for new spots on the skin that you haven't seen before, or spots that may be looking a little different compared to those around them, or a spot, mole or freckle that has changed in size, shape and colour, or even persistent sores that do not seem to be healing.

There's what we call the 'ABCDE' checklist for melanomas – it's easy to remember:

A – Alteration in appearance of a mole.

B – Borders changes/irregular border.

C – Colour changes.

D – Diameter greater than 6 mm.

E – Enlargement over a short period of time.

If you see changes or at least recognise one mole that might be increasing in size, you need to go and see your doctor and possibly get a referral to see a dermatologist to have it checked.

The DIY guide

Step 1 – Look at your face in the mirror, assessing your lips, mouth, nose, front and backs of ears, then your scalp (you may need someone else for this part).

Step 2 – Look at your hands and arms, assessing your fingernails, between the nails, the tops and bottoms of your hands, progressively working up the arms, remembering to check out the backs of your arms, the armpits and elbows.

Step 3 – Look at your neck, chest and stomach.

Step 4 – Check out your shoulders, your neck and down your spine.

Step 5 – Start looking from your waist to your toes. Assess both the front and backs of your legs, your lower legs, feet and toes. Look under the toenails, between the toes and under your feet.

The Cancer Council Australia recommends that if any spots on your body remain persistently dry and scale-like, go and seek further assessment from your doctor.

The professionals

Yeah, it's a pain going to the doctor – sometimes I think making the appointment is what puts people off, not the actual going-to-the-doctor part. If that's what's stopping you, ask someone else to make the appointment (I'm serious), then all you have to do is turn up. Because your GP is a good person to give your skin an initial check-up. He or she will look for any 'red flags', but if you have a family history of skin cancer or many moles and freckles they may recommend you see a dermatologist for follow-up. If your GP doesn't think anything's wrong but you're not so sure, never hesitate to get a second opinion. You're not going to offend anyone, and even if you did, it's worth it if you can either put your mind at ease or find out more information than you had before.

Skin cancer clinics are everywhere – in cities, at least – although they're not endorsed by the Cancer Council Australia at this stage, as many are private businesses run by GPs. Some clinics offer a higher level of expertise in skin examination compared with others, thus making it difficult for the Cancer Council to evaluate the care provided. Still, it can be hard to get an appointment with a GP, particularly if you've moved to a new area, so a skin cancer clinic is better than nothing.

You may be more inclined to use a skin cancer clinic because they bulk bill, so if you aren't sure whether or not to visit your nearest skin cancer clinic, the Cancer Council Australia recommend finding out about the expertise and professional background of the staff and what services they offer, the cost of the services, the diagnosis and treatment options available and the follow-up care provided.

If you have had previous skin cancer scares or you're at a higher risk – even if you just want a higher level of care – you're better off with a dermatologist. You should pay them a visit every twelve months for a routine check-up and they'll certainly give you a thorough going-over. It won't hurt, and it's worth the money if it keeps you in good nick. Not to press the analogy again, but you get your car serviced *at least* once a year, and you use your body more than your car. Just go to the doctor, orright?

The next step

If your doctor suspects you have a skin cancer, the first step is to take a biopsy. Depending on the size, location and appearance of the spot in question, this will be performed by your GP or by a specialist. This will generally require local anaesthetic – of course, Braveheart, you can try going without it – and a few stitches. In more extreme cases – and believe me, it's better to check often enough so that this never happens to you, unless you're fond of unconsciousness – it can be performed under a general anaesthetic.

The biopsy is tested to determine the type of cells affected, which decides the treatment options best suited to you.

Treatment options vary according to the type of cancer and whether it's likely to spread to other parts of the body. The options include:

- Surgery to remove the cancer, preventing further spread, and possibly to perform a skin graft over the effected site.
- A highly specialised surgical technique called 'Moh's Technique', which is used for difficult skin cancers.
- Cryotherapy – freezing and killing the cancer for its removal with liquid nitrogen.
- Curettage with cautery – a local anaesthetic is given at the site of the skin cancer, using a sharp instrument to scoop the cancer from the skin. An electric current is then used to destroy any possible tumour cells remaining.
- Imiquimod, which is a type of cream used to stimulate the body's immune system in order for the body to fight to destroy the cancer cells.
- Photodynamic therapy, which involves the use of a cream and light source to destroy cancer cells.
- Radiotherapy – using radiation treatment to kill cancer cells, normally over a period of weeks, targeting areas difficult for a surgeon to reach.
- Removal of lymph nodes – lymph nodes are used by the body to fight infection and foreign cells (such as cancerous cells). They're located in the neck, groin, pelvis, stomach and armpits. The removal of the lymph nodes protects you from the cancer spreading to other parts of your body.

Some of these options sound a little daunting, but the scarier ones are also the least common. As with all health problems, prevention is better than the cure – the earlier you get onto something, the less likely it is that you'll end up with radiotherapy or surgery. Moreover, you may have a BCC or SCC and not need either of those things. But you won't know whether you've got them – or nothing at all – if you don't check.

Protecting the duco every day of the year

We've had 'slip slop slap' and now we have cheerful TV ads showing surgeons operating on skin cancers. If we'd all paid more attention to the former campaign, maybe we wouldn't have needed the latter . . . I still think 'slip slop slap' is a great, simple message but in case you need a bit more detail.

1. Put on a broad-brimmed hat that shades your face and neck.
2. Wear sun-protective clothing that covers as much of your body as possible.
3. Seek shade whenever you are outdoors.
4. Wear wrap-around sunglasses.
5. Apply SPF30+ broad-spectrum water-resistant sunscreen every two hours.

Also, don't use solariums to get a tan – even if your girlfriend or boyfriend thinks you'll look better with one – and make sure you are out of the sun altogether between 11 a.m. and 3 p.m., the hottest part of the day. If you work outdoors this will be hard, so you'll need to take extra-special, extended-remix care of your skin.

Vitamin D and sun exposure

We all need vitamin D, which comes from the sun – but you only need sunlight for approximately ten minutes on most days of the week to receive adequate amounts of vitamin D from the sun and its UV rays in order to maintain healthy bones.

Generally, the amount of time you spend in the sun just getting from A to B is often adequate, if your arms, neck and face are exposed. In an interesting twist, a lack of vitamin D can impede your body's ability to fight cancer cells. The trick is in getting the balance right.

It's important to note that wearing sunscreen will prevent the absorption of vitamin D. So the best idea is to get your ten minutes early or late in the day, when the sun isn't so hot, and use sunscreen at other times.

Sunscreens

Sometimes I think buying sunscreen is so confusing for people that they give up and don't buy it at all. If this is you, I understand – but you still need to wear it. Some sunscreens are cheaper than others, some brands claim to have more protection than others – and there's all the differences in labelling. SPF 5, 10, 55, 2005 . . . argh!

According to Cancer Council Australia, the main role sunscreen plays in preventing skin cancer is limiting the amount of UV radiation being absorbed by the skin. Sunscreen can do this by either absorbing or reflecting UV radiation.

A sunscreen's label may say that the lotion is 'broad spectrum', which means the cream will protect the skin from both types of ultraviolet radiation, UVA and UVB radiation. UVA radiation affects the skin by causing wrinkles, discoloured areas, blotchiness and sagging, and it also heightens the risk of skin cancer. UVB radiation is mostly to blame for sunburns and causing the skin to tan.

There's usually also a spot on the label saying SPF, which stands for Sun Protection Factor. The SPF indicates the sunscreen's level of protection from UV radiation. The Cancer Council Australia recommends aiming for sunscreen with a 'Broad Spectrum SPF30+ water resistant' label, which should protect your skin from up to 97 per cent of UV radiation. You just have to make sure you're applying it properly and, most importantly, regularly. In terms of creams and sprays and lotions, use the type of sunscreen which is most appropriate to your activity. If you're going to sweat a lot, choose a sunscreen that doesn't wear off so easily.

If you're wondering whether the sunscreen you buy will be effective, rest assured: Australia has an effective Therapeutic Goods Administration, and every sunscreen sold is safe and effective. As to the cost; higher prices do not necessarily mean it is a better product. Quite often your choice will depend on the smell of the lotion – particularly if you're sensitive to fragrance – and how it feels on your skin. Test out sunscreens before you buy.

Most importantly before you buy, be sure to check the expiry date on the package. If the sunscreen is out of date, you might as well rub water into your skin.

It is now up to you to apply the sunscreen often enough to remain effective. Remember that sunscreen is never protecting you 100 per cent from the sun – you still need to cover yourself from the elements with shade, clothing, hats and sunglasses.

Sunscreen tips

According to the Cancer Council Australia, you will get optimal protection from your sunscreen if you:

- Apply sunscreen twenty minutes before you head outside.
- Use a generous amount of sunscreen over your body. On average, an adult should use up to 35 ml of sunscreen for one full-body application.
- Always reapply sunscreen every two hours when you are outdoors.
- Remember that when you sweat, sunscreen is easily wiped off so you need to keep putting sunscreen on to get the best protection.

Who does what

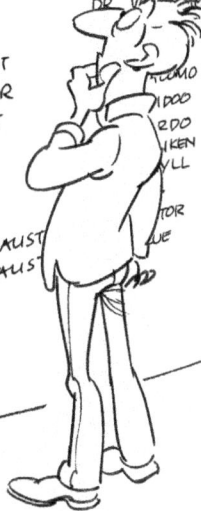

DR. SMITH
DR. ABRAHAMS
DR. MING
DR. ALEXANDER
DR. OLIPHANT
DR. HALL
DR. CULJAH
DR. WOODGATE
DR. MANSI
DR. MOTTOLA
DR. GIBSON
DR. RUNNALS
DR. CAPPILARI
DR. BEVAN
DR. GHANDI
DR. VERWOED
DR. NO
DR. BURTON
DR.

MEDICAL CENTRE

GENERAL PRACTITIONER DR. PAPAS
PROCTOLOGY   DR. CHANG
OBSTETRICS   DR. PAPADOPOULOS
OSTEOPATH   DR. CHENEY
GYNECOLOGY   DR BOFFA
PLASTIC SURGEON   DR. PIPER
DERMATOLOGY   DR. RICHARDS
ONCOLOGIST   DR.
PSYCHIATRY
ANAESTHETIST
CHIROPRACTOR
CARDIOLOGIST
HOMEOPATH
DRALOGIST
PSYCHIATRY
OSTEOPATH
BEAUTY SPECIALIST
UGLY SPECIALIST

GERIATRICS
PATHOLOGIST
NEURO SURGEON
MAMMOGRAPHY
HAEMOTOLOGY
PHARMOCOLOGY
PAEDIATRICS
NEPHROLOGY
G.P.
RADIOLOGY
PERIODONTIST
CARDIOLOGY
TOXICOLOGY
PATHOLOGY
ROADOLOGY
ANYTHING.
TAUTOLOGY
COLOURIST.

General practitioners

General practitioners (GPs) are generally considered – by civilians and governments alike – to be the first port of call when you have a health concern. It is up to the GP to identify the problem; if they can't help you they need to refer you on to a health professional who *can* help. This other health professional may be a medical specialist or a health worker such as an occupational therapist, physiotherapist or dietitian or nutritionist. Your GP is not meant to be able to fix everything for you as the name suggests, he or she is a *general* practitioner and does not have specialist knowledge.

The health problems GPs commonly see include those related to injuries, illness, sexual health, contraception, emotional issues, depression, nutrition problems, relaxation, immunisations, blood collecting and health checks.

First of all it's important to actually have a GP – not just whoever is on rotation at your local 24-hour medical centre, but a live human being who has your medical records on hand. These days it's not always possible to find one of these quasi-unicorns – country and city dwellers alike are affected by the GP shortage – so a medical centre can suffice *if absolutely necessary*.

If you do have a GP, it's important to feel comfortable with them and their abilities. If you're not quite sure, get a second opinion – there may be another doctor in the same practice that you can see. Follow your own 'gut instinct' about your health – if you reckon that your doctor hasn't quite nailed the diagnosis, then go with that feeling. It can't hurt to get a second opinion, but it may hurt a whole lot if you don't.

Casualty/emergency

An important point to note is that the casualty or emergency ward of your local hospital is *not* a general practice. Please do not waltz up there with a sniffle or an ear ache, unless you suspect there's a baby cockroach living on your ear drum – and, even then, a GP can probably get it out. Hospital resources are stretched at the best of times and need to be saved for people with genuine emergencies – burns, bleeding, internal injuries. Your sprained ankle is not in this category. Get thee to a GP.

Dentists

It staggers me how many people don't see a dentist regularly. Are you MAD? You only get one set of teeth! Look after them! Just like the rest of your body, teeth benefit from regular check-ups and good caretaking. Your dentist can take care of the first part. If you haven't been to a dentist for years, ask around your friends for a recommendation. There's absolutely no need to be afraid, and even if you're worried about your dentist coming at you with a large drill, don't fret – they have good drugs to help you through that stuff.

Specialists

Now we come to the specialists – the people your GP should refer you to as needed. This list is just an indication of the type of professional you may need to see, to help you familiarise yourself with the terms. Of course, your regular doctor will be able to give you a specific referral.

The Problem	The Expert
Adrenal gland problems	Endocrinologist
Allergies or immune problems	Immunologist
Ankle injuries	Sports medicine specialist

Anti-ageing therapies	Plastic/reconstructive specialist or plastic surgeon
Arthritic problems	Rheumatologist
Babies' health	Paediatrician
Back pain/injury	Physiotherapist
Bladder problem	Urologist
Blood problems	Haematologist
Brain problems	Neurologist
Cancer	Oncologist
Chronic fatigue	Rheumatologist
Cleft lip and palate	Plastic/reconstructive specialist or plastic surgeon
Cosmetic surgery	Plastic reconstructive specialist or plastic surgeon
CT scan	Radiologist
Diabetes	Endocrinologist
Ear, nose and throat problems	Ear, nose and throat (ENT) specialist
Eye problems	Ophthalmologist
Facelift and eyelids	Plastic/reconstructive Specialist or plastic surgeon
Fibromyalgia	Rheumatologist
Foot injuries	Sports medicine specialist
Gallbladder problems	Gastroenterologist or general surgeon
General anaesthetic	Anaesthetist

General issues – laparoscopic, obesity, gallbladder, and the list goes on . . .	General surgeon
Hand surgery	Plastic/reconstructive specialist or plastic surgeon
Head and neck surgery	Plastic/reconstructive specialist or plastic surgeon
Heartburn	Gastroenterologist
Heart problem	Cardiologist
Infectious diseases	Infectious diseases specialist
Jaundice	Gastroenterologist
Kids' health	Paediatrician
Kidney stones/problems	Urologist
Knee injuries	Sports medicine specialist
Lithotripsy	Urologist
Liver problems	Gastroenterologist
Lung problems	Respiratory specialist
Mental health problems	Psychiatrist/Psychologist
Mouth or facial problems	Oral/maxillofacial specialist
MRI Scan	Radiologist
Musculoskeletal injuries	Sports medicine specialist
Nose job (rhinoplasty)	Plastic/reconstructive specialist or plastic surgeon
Oesophagus problems	Gastroenterologist
Old age problems	Geriatrician
Pancreas problems	Gastroenterologist
Pineal gland problems	Endocrinologist

Pituitary problems	Endocrinologist
Prostate problems	Urologist
Reconstructive surgery	Plastic/reconstructive specialist or plastic surgeon
Rectal bleeding	Gastroenterologist
Rehabilitation from injury and pain issues	Physical/rehabilitation specialist
Skin problems	Dermatologist
Skeletal/bone problems	Orthopaedic specialist/ orthopaedist (surgeon)
Skin cancer	Plastic/reconstructive specialist or plastic surgeon
Skin treatments	Plastic/reconstructive specialist or plastic surgeon
Stomach and bowel problems	Gastroenterologist
Thyroid and parathyroid	Endocrinologist
Ultrasound	Radiologist
Urinary/genitourinary problems	Urologist
Vasectomy	Urologist
Women's health	Gynaecologist and/or obstetrician
X-ray	Radiologist

Glossary

Here is a list of medical terms you might come across in your travels. Remember: Ask your doctor to explain if you don't understand the jargon.

Acne Commonly seen in teenage years at the onset of and during puberty; a result of inflammation of the sebaceous glands.

Anejaculation No ejaculation at all. Semen is unable to travel from the prostate or seminal ducts into the urethra.

Anorgasmia You're unable to achieve an orgasm.

Alzheimer's disease Progressive neurological condition affecting parts of the brain, slowly changing the individual's personality, memory and thinking. Occurs in both men and women and is also linked to genes (i.e. hereditary). Common symptoms include confusion, poor memory, difficulty making simple decisions, appearing irritated. Slowly symptoms become worse and the sufferer possibly forgets places/occasions/family names/friends, can no longer focus on a conversation, is no longer able to care for their house and even themselves, and experiences loss of speech. Often the sufferer ends up in a nursing home needing full-time care by nurses.

Anaesthetic A special drug that prevents a person from feeling pain during a medical procedure. Local anaesthetic directly numbs a part of the body, whereas a general anaesthetic given by a trained anaesthetic doctor (anaesthetist) causes a person to lose consciousness throughout the length of a surgical procedure.

Arrhythmia Abnormal heart rhythm and abnormal heart rate.

Arthritis Swollen (inflamed) joint.

Apnoea Breathing stops for a few seconds to up to a minute

Atrium Upper chamber of the heart, both left and right side. Collects blood from the body, pumping the blood into the ventricles toward the body.

Asynchrony Heart rhythm is not in sequence when the heart chambers contract.

Basal cell cancer A type of skin cancer affecting the basal cells of the top layer of the skin (epidermis).

Benign Not cancerous or malignant, therefore not able to spread (metastasise) like cancer cells.

Biopsy The removal of abnormal tissue from the body. The sample is examined under a microscope, allowing the specialist to diagnose the disease or type of cells affected.

Bradycardia Slow pulse or heartbeat, considered to be anything under 60 beats per minute.

Bunions An enlarged portion of the joint near the big toe (most commonly). It forms when the toes move out of place. When the big toe moves towards the other toes the bunion grows. (In Latin bunion means 'enlargement'.)

Bursitis Inflammation of the sac of synovial fluid (bursa) located around joints

Cancer A disease of the body's cells. Disease or damage to the cells cause abnormal cells to form and they can start to multiply, forming a growth or a tumour.

Cardiac arrest The heart muscle stops beating completely or the heart beats so fast it is unable to pump sufficient blood around the body.

Cardioversion A low to moderate amount of energy used to give electrical shock to a person reverting an abnormal heart rhythm to a normal heart rhythm (sinus rhythm).

Cautery A type of treatment used for skin cancer. This technique uses an electrical current to destroy the tissue.

Circadian rhythm The word circadian refers to a one-day cycle. Circadian rhythm is programmed to work over a set 24-hour period. When you experience sunlight this instantly sends messages to the brain's neurotransmitters, prompting your body to coordinate bodily functions. It affects sleep, body temperature, energy levels, libido, the amount of hormones released, your blood pressure, heart rate, mood and digestion.

Clubfoot Otherwise known as talipes. It's a deformity present at birth, commonly in a bone in the ankle (talus). The foot appears to point down and is twisted in at the ankle. The foot appears smaller than usual, the joints stiffened and the calf muscle is often smaller too. The condition does not correct itself – it must be treated.

Colonoscopy This term refers to the use of a scope (camera) to view the colon.

Congestive heart failure (CHF) A weakened heart muscle prevents the heart from pumping effectively in order to supply the body with enough blood. This is caused by too much fluid being 'congested' within the heart and surrounding blood vessels, which basically makes it very hard for blood and bodily fluids to move around the body. This congestion can cause extra fluid (oedema) to build up in areas of the body, such as the legs, the lungs and the abdomen, causing the person to look puffy. It's caused by uncontrolled high blood pressure, heart disease and cardiomyopathy. Symptoms include feeling breathless while not doing much; feeling tired; swollen ankles; weak pulse but beating rapidly; low blood pressure; pale skin; swelling around the stomach; tired muscles; coughing and wheezing for no reason.

Continuous Positive Airway Pressure (CPAP) This is used for people with obstructive sleep apnoea. A pump delivers a set pressure of air through a long hose-like tube to a mask, positioned either over your nose or your face, which you wear whenever you sleep – night/day/naps. The machine forces positive pressure through your nose or mouth into the back of your throat, ensuring it remains open, allowing air to reach your lungs while you are sleeping. Generally CPAP is used for those with moderate to severe sleep apnoea.

Cryotherapy A type of treatment used for skin cancer. This technique destroys tissue by using extreme cold liquid, known as liquid nitrogen.

Curettage Removal of small growths using a spoon-shaped instrument with a sharp edge, called a curette.

Defibrillation Delivery of an electrical shock to the chest/heart, in order to return a dangerous heart rhythm back to a normal heart rhythm (sinus rhythm).

Defibrillator A machine able to deliver the required amounts of electrical energy to the heart to change a life-threatening (too fast and irregular) heart rhythm to a normal heart rhythm (sinus rhythm). This is delivered to the person using paddles or pads applied to the chest.

Delayed ejaculation When an extreme amount of arousal is needed to have an orgasm with ejaculation.

Dementia A decline in normal brain function.

Dermatologist A doctor who is a specialist in the prevention, diagnosis and treatment of skin problems.

Dermis The dermis is the second layer of the skin. The epidermis sits above the dermis.

Diabetes A condition in which a person's pancreas is not producing insulin or is producing insufficient amounts of insulin in the body, in order to convert sugar (glucose) from food into energy.

Dysplastic naevus A mole with irregular shape and various colours.

Dyslexia Otherwise refered to as a specific learning disorder. A person has difficulty recognising words, spelling or writing, generally having trouble with language. Symptoms might include avoiding reading or writing wherever possible and evident problems with reading and spelling.

ECG (Electrocardiogram) A graph depicting the heart's electrical signals and flow of impulses throughout the heart, from twelve different views. The graph is printed on paper, allowing the medical and nursing team to read your heart rhythm. The test takes about ten minutes.

Ejection fraction The percentage of blood pumped or ejected from the left side of your heart (left ventricle) with each beat towards the rest of the body.

Epidermis One of two main layers that make up the skin. The epidermis is the top or outer layer (see also dermis).

Electrophysiology Study (EPS) A test looking at the electrical signals in your heart. The test helps to identify and diagnose abnormal heart rhythms in people, as well as the problem areas and what treatment options are best for the person The EPS is also useful in testing that a pacemaker already inside the person is working to the best of its ability.

Fatigue Ongoing feeling of tiredness, both mental and physical

Faecal Occult Blood Test (FOBT) A screening tool for bowel cancer. The test can be done in your own home. You place two or three consecutive stool specimens into a container in order to send to a pathology lab for testing, assessing for potential risk of bleeding within the bowel.

Gastroscopy Use of a scope to check the small bowel. The camera goes down the mouth into the gastrointestinal system – oesophagus, stomach and small bowel.

Gestational diabetes This affects women only during their pregnancy or for a short period after the delivery.

Gout A very common problem among you fellas. It refers to an inflammation of any joint of the body, most often affecting the big toe joint (first metatarsophalangeal joint). The initial attack will come on suddenly (overnight), accompanied by swelling and severe pain to the joint. Attacks may vary from months to years, but become more frequent over time. The skin over the joint can become shiny in appearance.

Heart attack Otherwise known as a myocardial infarction (MI). The name literally means 'heart muscle death' so, basically, not enough blood flow to an area of the heart will cause muscle death. It's often caused by a blocked artery in the heart. Warning signs include pain in the chest, upper jaw, arm, shoulder blade, neck, nausea, and possible shortness of breath.

Heartbeat You may know this as pulse or heart rate. It refers to the pumping action and cycle of all four chambers in the heart, allowing the heart to pump blood to the rest of the body.

Heart block Signifies that the heart's electrical impulses are not flowing through the heart as intended – they are blocked or delayed for some reason. This can cause your heart to 'skip a beat'.

Heartburn Otherwise known as reflux. It feels like a burning in your food pipe (oesophagus) in the area of your chest and is considered to be a form of indigestion. The chewed food, combined with stomach acids, is forced back into the oesophagus, causing the burning sensation. Heartburn is caused by a variety of things such as anxiety, being overweight, eating large meals and lying down soon afterwards, drinking a lot of coffee or alcohol or taking specific medications, end-stage pregnancy, slouching after eating big meals, and hiatus hernia.

Heart failure Failure of the heart muscle to pump effectively, supplying the body with enough blood around the body. (See also Congestive Heart Failure.)

Heart murmur Abnormal heart sounds caused by leaking heart valves or narrowed valves, heart disorders, stress or sometimes anaemia. You can often have no symptoms and it may not affect your health.

Heart rhythm Otherwise known as a pulse or heartbeat, signifying the speed and regularity of the beat. Normal heart rate is considered to be between 60 to 100 beats per minute while resting.

Herniated disc Otherwise known as a slipped disc. The soft, spongy part between each vertebra within the intervertebral disc is ruptured, protruding out of the disc, this can be bloody painful to say the least, resulting in nerve pain in the back and legs.

Hyperglycaemia A condition caused by high levels of glucose in the blood

Hypoglycaemia Blood glucose levels drop too low, causing you to feel a little shaky or almost faint.

Implantable Cardioverter Defibrillator (ICD) You may know this as a defib pacemaker. The device is similar to a pacemaker, as it monitors and helps to maintain your heartbeat, but it helps to treat the heart rhythm if it is beating dangerously too fast or too slow.

Keratoses Also known as sunspots. They look like flat, scaly areas on the skin and are the result of sun damage to the skin.

Ketoacidosis This occurs when a diabetic (mostly type 1) does not have enough insulin in the body, and this then causes the blood glucose levels to grow extremely high. Rather then the body using glucose for energy it starts using body fat for energy instead. the condition is highly toxic for the body.

Lyme disease A disease caused by a bacterium (*Borrelia burgdorferi*) transmitted via ticks. It can cause headaches, stiff joints, fever, chills, nausea, lower back pain and a stiff neck.

Lymph nodes Also known as lymph glands. Small bean-shaped lymph cells clumped together along the lymphatic system. Their job in the body is to get rid of bacteria and other little foreign pests. They are predominantly located in the neck, armpit, groin and abdomen.

Malignant This means that a tumour is cancerous. These types of cells can spread (metastasise), affecting other parts of the body, which if not treated, can cause death.

Melanin The pigment that gives skin its colour. It can protect the body against the damaging effect of ultraviolet (UV) rays.

Melanocytes Cells that produce melanin, located in the top layer of the skin (epidermis).

Melanoma Cancer of the melanocytes. A dangerous form of skin cancer which can also affect your mouth and nasal passage. UV radiation can cause melanoma.

Menopause Is the term given when there has been an absence of menstrual periods for twelve consecutive months.

Metabolism Takes into account all of the chemical processes within the body, looking at both the input and output of energy. It also regulates the amount of energy your body burns.

Metastases Commonly referred to as 'secondaries'. Malignant tumour cells can break away from the primary (initial) cancer and start affecting other parts of the body, causing secondary cancers.

Mohs technique A specialised surgical procedure using microscopic equipment in order to remove skin cancers one segment at a time until only normal cells remain.

Myocardial infarction See heart attack.

Naevi You would know these as 'moles'. They come from melanocytes.

Obstructive sleep apnoea A condition which occurs when a person sleeps, causing them to stop breathing for a few seconds to up to a minute at a time as a result of an obstructed airway.

Osteoporosis A condition resulting in weakened bones (decreased bone mass) increasing the risk of breaking (fracturing) your bones. It occurs when bones lose calcium (and other minerals) at a rate faster then it can be replaced. Commonly affects bones in the hip, spine, wrist, upper arm, ribs, and pelvis. Often associated with postmenopause (oestrogen deficiency); it can be age related (bone loss as a result of ageing); diet-related (chronic dietary deficiency in calcium and protein, and Vitamin C); disuse and genes.

Paget's disease A disorder of the bone resulting in abnormal thickening and softening of the bone, due to accelerated bone growth. What causes this is still not understood. Common bones affected include the skull, spine, pelvis, and the long bones of the arm and thigh.

Painful ejaculation Pain around the perineum, groin or in the urethra during an erection. Often due to a blockage or swelling in the area.

Painful heel syndrome The fancy name is plantar fasciitis and it refers to inflammation around the heel bone as a result of long-term irritation to the fascia (the membrane responsible for separating, covering and supporting muscles). Often due to overuse and continuous impact of running and walking.

Pathologist A pathologist is a specialist doctor who examines tissue samples (biopsies) under a microscope to diagnose cancer and other diseases.

Photodynamic therapy (PDT) A treatment technique used for skin cancers using the combination of light source and a special cream to destroy cancer cells.

Placenta Otherwise known as the afterbirth, this is delivered after the baby is born. This unique organ allows the foetus to gain nourishment during the nine months of pregnancy through the exchange of bodily fluids between mother and foetus, also allowing waste products from the foetus to be passed onto the mother in order to exit the body.

Perforation Another word for 'tearing'.

Peri-menopause This refers to the time around menopause. It is very different for each woman and can begin ten years before the official last period.

Polyp The growth of tissue found in various areas of the body.

Post-menopause The time after the last menstrual period. In other words, the rest of a woman's life after the last menstrual period.

Pre-diabetes Otherwise known as impaired glucose metabolism, basically pre-diabetes is an indication of the blood glucose levels being a little too high to be normal, yet not high enough to be diabetes.

Prognosis A doctor may explain a prognosis to you after being told you have a specific disease such as cancer. A prognosis assesses the course and possible outcome of the disease or cancer.

Radiotherapy The use of radiation to kill cancer cells preventing further growth or spread within the body. Radiotherapy treatment can also harm normal cells, but ideally this will affect a limited number of cells which are then able to repair themselves.

Retrograde ejaculation Semen actually travels backwards to the bladder rather than out via the urethra. The urine often looks cloudy after sex due to mixing with the semen.

Rheumatism Often referred to as arthritis, osteoarthritis, bursitis and sciatica. It refers to painful states of inflammation and breakdown of connective tissue occurring in the bones, ligaments, joints, tendons and muscles.

Sciatica Swelling (inflammation) of to the sciatic nerve. This nerve runs down the backs of the thigh towards the inside of the leg, sending pain from the back to the legs, feet and possibly toes. Sciatic pain can be caused by injury or inflammation to the sciatic nerve, slipped or herniated discs, back injuries, diabetes mellitus, irritation due to arthritis of the spine, gout, and vitamin deficiencies.

Secondary Otherwise known as metastasis. A growth or tumour may spread from the original cancer site to another part of the body, causing further cancerous growths.

Shingles Caused by the *varicella zoster* virus (responsible for the chickenpox), otherwise known as *herpes zoster*, causing an acute infection to the peripheral nervous system (basically the engine which controls all the nerves of the body). Shingles develops as a rash, mostly to one side of the body/trunk or to the face and is considered to be quite painful. The virus lies dormant in the body, sitting at the base of the nerve cells which allow sensations to the skin. The virus can suddenly become active again, causing very painful sensations to the nerves of the affected area, multiplying and spreading rapidly along the nerves. A person can develop shingles only if they have had chickenpox previously. You can catch chickenpox from another person who at that time is infected with either chickenpox or shingles.

Skin graft Under surgical intervention, a piece of healthy skin is removed from one part of the body and transferred to another area on the body in order to cover and help heal a wound.

Skin cancer Generalised description of various malignant tumours that occur within the epidermal cells. Common skin cancers include basal cell carcinoma, squamous cell carcinoma and malignant melanoma.

Smelly feet Our feet have many sweat glands, which work

overtime when we're hot, stressed, busy, experiencing hormonal changes or as a result of taking certain drugs. When we cover our feet with a hot sock and a non-airing boot, and that's combined with thriving bacteria, we soon develop a unique whofting smell. Apparently the bacteria produces isovaleric acid, which causes the odour.

Sprain Forced twisting of a joint (commonly ankles or wrists) with a degree of swelling and damage to ligaments, with possible injury to blood vessels, nerves, muscles and tendons without dislocating the joint.

Squamous cell cancer Skin cancer affecting the squamous cells in the top layer of the skin.

Strain Overstretching of a muscle without the swelling, often as a result of overexercising.

Stroke Otherwise known as a CVA (cerebral vascular attack/cerebrovascular attack). A stroke is caused by damage or narrowing to the blood vessels in the brain to the point where the person is not getting enough blood (with oxygen) to the brain, causing partial death (infarction) to the brain tissue. If the left brain is affected then it is the right side of the body which may become paralysed, causing difficulties with speech and memory along with slow behavioural changes. If the right brain is affected then it is the left side of the body which may become paralysed, causing difficulties with perception and also memory with quick impulsive changes to the person's behaviour.

Testicular torsion What happens when a testis (it generally only ever happens to one at a time) twists from its tube (the spermatic cord), potentially cutting off blood supply to the testis.

TIA Refers to transient ischemic attack, otherwise known as a 'mini stroke'. This is caused by interrupted blood flow to areas of the brain affecting the neurological function for short periods of time.

Tumour Abnormal growth of tissue on or in the body.

Ultraviolet (UV) radiation The part of sunlight that causes the skin to burn, causing prolonged damage. Also present in solariums, tanning lamps and sun beds.

UV Index This is a measurement of the sun's UV radiation and it's intensity.

Ventricle One of the two lower chambers of the heart. The ventricle receives blood from the upper half of the heart, the atria; the right ventricle pumps blood into the lungs and the left ventricle pumps oxygenated blood to the body.

Ventricular fibrillation (VF) This is an irregular heart rhythm which beats very fast, limiting the amount of blood the heart can pump for the rest of the body. VF can cause the heart to beat up to 300 beats per minute, way too fast. A defibrillator is required to change the electrical impulses to a normal regular beating rhythm. This rhythm can be fatal.

Ventricular tachycardia (VT) Caused by abnormal electrical impulses, which make the heart beat very fast. VT can cause the heart to beat 120 to 250 beats per minute. A defibrillator is required to change the electrical impulses, to a normal regular beating rhythm. This rhythm can be fatal.

Your own personal log book

Problem	Test(s)	Routine Check	Family History
High Blood Pressure (BP)	BP	– If normal every 6 to 12 months unless advised otherwise by your doctor. – More frequent if newly diagnosed. – More frequent if changing medication. – More frequent if losing weight.	Inform GP
Slow Pulse	BP + Heart Rate + ECG	– Take your pulse, count how many beats per minute. – Normal is 60 to 100 bpm. – Discuss with GP.	Inform GP

Problem	Test(s)	Routine Check	Family History
Chest Pain	BP + ECG Bloods tests	**Call 000** Seek immediate medical attention.	
Prostate	PSA	– If no relevant symptoms first one at 50 years of age. – If you have family history get checked at 40 years of age. – If problems with waterworks see your GP.	Inform GP
	DRE	– If no relevant symptoms first one at 50 years of age. – If you have family history get checked at 40 years of age. – If problems with your waterworks see your GP.	Inform GP
Bowel Health	FOBT	– If no relevant symptoms start checking at 50 years of age.	Inform GP of any bowel health history.

Problem	Test(s)	Routine Check	Family History
	Colonoscopy + Endoscopy	– If one of your family members had/has polyps or bowel cancer commence diagnostic screening 10 years prior to the age your relative was diagnosed. – Your specialist may require you to continue with repeat scopes every 2 to 5 years.	
Testicles	Self-examination	– First Monday of each month.	Inform GP if this is in your family.
	Medical Assessment	– If lumps, swelling or other concerns.	
Skin Check	Self-examination	– Every 3 months from scalp to soles.	Inform GP
	Skin clinic or Dermatologist	– Every 12 months if results normal.	

Problem	Test(s)	Routine Check	Family History
Obesity	Waist Measurement	– Every few months to ensure your belly is less than 94 cm with a simple tape measure.	If you know you are at risk make lifestyle changes early before it becomes a problem.
Teeth	Brush & Floss	– Brush teeth morning & night. – Floss daily.	Does not have to be your problem too.
	Visit your dentist	– Every 6 months.	
Impotence	Physical Examination; Medical history	– See your GP if there is a problem or it's not performing like it normally does.	
Premature Ejacu- lation	Physical Examination; Medical history;	– See your GP if this is a new problem or your performance is 'not normal' for you.	

Problem	Test(s)	Routine Check	Family History
Diabetes	Blood Glucose Level (BGL)	– If you are a diag-nosed 'Diabetic' you may have to take your BGL twice or even up to 4 times per day. – Your GP, specialist or diabetic educator will let you know what you need to do.	Inform GP
	Blood Test	– To diagnose diabetes, or to ensure your BGL are being controlled properly.	

Abbreviations

PSA   Prostate Specific Antigen
DRE   Digital Rectal Examination
FOBT   Faecal Occult Blood Test
ECG   Electrocardiogram

Bibliography

Ageing Well, The Jean Hailes Foundation for Women's Health, www.ageingwell.org.au

Ashfield J, 2007, *Taking Care of Yourself and Your Family, A Resource Book for Good Mental Health*, Peacock Publications, Australia. Available from www.beyondblue.org.au (accessed August 2008)

Arthritis Australia, www.arthritisaustralia.com.au

Australian Bureau of Statistics 2004–05. Available from www.abs.gov.au

Australian Bureau of Statistics, 2006, *National Health Survey 2004 – 2005 Summary of Results*. Available from: www.abs.gov.au

Australian Government National Health and Medical Research Council, *Hormone Replacement Therapy: Exploring the Options for Women*, March 2005

Australian Institute of Health and Welfare, 2006, *Australia's Health 2006*, AIHW Cat. No. AUS 73, AIHW, Canberra. Available from www.aihw.gov.au (accessed November 2008)

Australasian College of Skin Cancer Medicine. Available from www.skincancercollege.com/Home/Patient_info/Treatment/PDT. aspx (accessed February 2009)

Bartlett, DJ, Paisley, L, Desai, AV, 2006, 'Insomnia Diagnosis and

Management', *Medicine Today* August 2006, Vol 7, No. 8

Better Health Channel, http://www.betterhealth.vic.gov.au

BeyondBlue, www.beyondblue.org.au

Black Dog Institute, www.blackdoginstitute.org.au

Borushek A, 2008, *Allan Borushek's Calorie, Fat and Carbohydrate Counter*, Family Health Publications, Western Australia

Bowel Cancer and Digestive Research Institute Australia, http://www.itscrunchtime.org

Bowel Cancer and Digestive Research Institute Australia, Media Release, 'Simple, inexpensive test to screen for bowel cancer risk', 5 March 2008. Available from http://www.itscrunchtime.org (accessed August 2008)

Brand-Miller J, Foster-Powell K, Colagiuri S, Barclay A, 2007, *The New Glucose Revolution, Diabetes and Pre-Diabetes Handbook*, Hachette, Australia

Brand-Miller J, Foster-Powell K, McMillan-Price J, 2004, *The Low GI Diet*, Hodder, Australia

Brand-Miller J, Farid NR, Marsh K, 2004, *The New Glucose Revolution Managing PCOS*, Hodder, Australia

Buscemi N, Vandermeer B, Pandya R, et al. *Melatonin for Treatment of Sleep Disorders. Summary, Evidence, Report/Technology Assessment*: Number 108. AHRQ Publication Number 05-E002-1, November 2004. Agency for Healthcare Research & Quality, Rockville, MD, http://www.ahrq.gov/clinic/epcsums/melatsum.htm

Campbell-McBride N, 2004, *Gut and Psychology Syndrome*, Medinform, United Kingdom

Cancer Institute NSW, 2007, *Melanoma Fact Sheet*. Available from http://www.cancerinstitute.org.au/cancer_inst/publications/pdfs/2008-01-18_melanoma.pdf (accessed 12 December 2008)

Cancer Institute NSW, http://www.cancerinstitute.org.au

Cabot S, 1991, *Menopause, Hormone Replacement Therapy and Its Natural Alternatives*, WHAS, Australia

Channel 9 News, 'Bowel cancer knowledge "alarmingly low"', 12 February, 2008. Available from http://news.ninemsn.com.au/article.aspx?id=67515 (accessed 12 February 2008)

Darovic GO, 2002, *Hemodynamic Monitoring Invasive and Noninvasive Clinical Application*, 3rd edition, W.B. Saunders Company, US

Department of Ageing, Disability & Home Care, http://www.dadhc.nsw.gov.au

Grunstein, RR, 'Obstructive Sleep Apnoea – Getting to the Heart of the Matter?' *Medical Journal of Australia 2008*; 188 (6):324–325. Available from http://www.mja.com.au/public/issues/188_06_170308/gru11260_fm (accessed March 2008)

Hall L, 'Don't blame Joey for illness says doctor'. Sun-Herald, 2 September 2007. Available from www.leaguehq.com.au/news/news/dont-blame-joey-for-illness-says-doctor/2007/09/01/1188067439139.html

Health Network, 2005, *Premature Ejaculation*. Available from http://www.healthnetwork.com.au/men/premature-ejaculation.asp (accessed October 2008)

Health Network, 2005, *Penis Enlargement*. Available from http://www.healthnetwork.com.au/men/penis-enlargement.asp (accessed October 2008)

Heart Foundation, 2007, Media Release, 'Newspoll reveals 56 per cent of people in NSW would not call an ambulance when experiencing heart attack warning signs', 30 April.

Heart Foundation, 2007, *Blood Pressure Facts*. Available from www.heartfoundation.com.au (accessed November 2007)

Heart Foundation, 2004, *Statistics*. Available from www.heartfoundation.org.au/Heart_Information/Statistics.htm

Hunter New England NSW Health, May 2005, *A-Z Health Topics*, Media Release – 'Still the Number One Killer'. Available from www.hnehealth.nsw.gov.au/news/releases/2005/May/heart_cardiovascular.html (accessed November 2007)

Impotence Australia, http://www.ImpotenceAustralia.com.au

JobAccess – An Australian Government Initiative, *Gout Information*, 12 December, 2008. Available from www.jobaccess.gov.au/JOAC/Advice/DisabilityOne/Gout.htm (accessed 20 December 2008)

Kennedy, GA, Bruck, D., Date unknown, *Sleep Disorders*, NSW Central West Division of General Practice GP Mental Health Supplement

Kick, K, 1997, *Adult Nursing Acute and Community Care*, 2nd edition, p. 1751

Kowalski R.E., 2006, *Take The Pressure Off Your Heart*, New Holland, Australia

Leigh B, 2007, *Men Surviving Cancer*, Jane Curry Publishing, Australia

Llewellyn-Jones, D, 1993, *Everywoman – A Gynaecological Guide For Life*, Penguin, pp 7–10

McMahon CG, *New Drugs, Old Drugs, Erectile Dysfunction*, MJA 2000; 173:492-497

Menopause Centre, www.menopausecentre.com.au

MenSheds Australia, www.menssheds.com.au

Mensline, www.mensline.org.au

Milham C, *Australian Healthy Shopping Guide*, 2007, Starbust Publishing, Australia

Miller-Keane, 1997, Encyclopedia and Dictionary of Medicine, Nursing & Allied Health, 6th Edition, Saunders, US

National Bowel Cancer Screening Program, www.cancerscreening.gov.au

National Heart Foundation, October 2007, *Heart Facts: Cardiovascular Disease Men and Women*, Available from www.heartfoundation.org.au (accessed 15 December 2008)

National Sleep Foundation, 2005, 'Danger on the Road? Sleep Apnoea High Amongst Truck Drivers', Vol. 7, Issue 1 of *Sleepmatters* Magazine. Available from www.sleepfoundation.org (accessed June 2008)

National Sleep Foundation, 2005, Drowsy Driving, Available from www.sleepfoundation.org (accessed June 2008)

NSW Health, *A-Z Health Topics – Cardiovascular Disease*. Available from www.health.nsw.gov.au/topics/cardiovascular.html (accessed November 2007)

Nutrition Australia, 1992, *The Australian Calorie Counter*, Penguin, Australia

Osiecki H, 2006, *The Physician's Handbook of Clinical Nutrition*, 7th Edition, Australia, AG Publishing

Palmer & Stuckey, 'Premature Ejaculation: a clinical update', *Medical Journal of Australia*, June 2008; Vol.188, No.11: 662-666 Available from www.mja.com.au/public/issues/188_11_020608/pal11233_fm.html (accessed November 2008)

Prostate Cancer Foundation of Australia, www.prostate.org.au

Sleep Disorders Australia, 2007, *CPAP* Brochure. Available from www.sleepoz.org.au (accessed February 2008)

Sleep Disorders Australia, 2006, *Delayed Sleep Phase Syndrome* Brochure. Available from www.sleepoz.org.au (accessed February 2008)

Sleep Disorders Australia, 2006, *Drowsy Driving* Brochure. Available from www.sleepoz.org.au (accessed February 2008)

Sleep Disorders Australia, 2007, *Sleep Apnoea* Brochure. Available from www.sleepoz.org.au (accessed February 2008)

Sleep Disorders Australia, 2007, *Sleep Study* Brochure. Available from www.sleepoz.org.au (accessed February 2008)

Sleep Disorders Australia, 2007, *Snoring* Brochure, Available from www.sleepoz.org.au (accessed February 2008)

The Australian Lung Foundation, www.lungnet.com.au

The Cancer Council NSW, 2007, *Understanding Prostate Cancer: A Guide for Men with Cancer, Their Families and Friends*

The Cancer Council NSW, 2007, *Understanding Testicular Cancer: A Guide for Men with Cancer, Their Families and Friends*

The Cancer Council NSW, www.cancercouncil.com.au

The Cancer Council Australia, www.cancer.org.au

The Gut Foundation, www.gut.nsw.edu.au/pcinfo4.htm#cancer

Tortora GJ, Grabowski SR, 1996, *Principles of Anatomy and Physiology*, 8th Edition, HarperCollins, US

Whitney EN, Cataldo CB, Rolfes SR, 2002, *Understanding Normal and Clinical Nutrition*, 6th Edition, Wadsworth, US

Index

Acknowledgments

Thank you to my dear mum and dad for your encouragement and belief in my ambitions and vision. You have always instilled in me to follow my passion and never give up. I thank you and love you both dearly! I would also like to thank the rest of my family, most importantly my two brothers, Scott and Mark, who have also shown endless encouragement and support throughout this process – and yes, I did take many of those sarcastic remarks as encouragement (as only sisters do)!

In recognition of a significant turning point, I would like to acknowledge a very dear mate, Nick Gibson, whose death changed my life. Nick passed away at the age of 32 in 2006 from a spontaneous brain aneurysm. It was the senseless loss of his life that made me realise life is so very precious, that we need to embrace it with both hands and make a difference. If we have a dream, we must follow it through. Six weeks after Nick's death I left my job and decided to pursue the dream I had been mapping for the previous three years. I started studying a diploma of nutrition while I worked part time as a nurse, before starting to give my talks in workplaces. Nick, I thank you for your friendship, your inspiration and your passion for life. I wish you were still here with James and all of us.

A very big thank you to the team at Hachette Australia, especially Vanessa and Sandy, who gave me this wonderful opportunity. Vanessa, thank you for your ongoing guidance.

I would like to thank the following doctors for their time in proofing the earlier drafts of the book: Dr Keith Kelly (anaesthetic specialist);

Dr Simon Benstock (gastroenterologist); Dr Cameron Bell (gastroenterologist and boardmember of the Bowel Cancer and Digestive Research Institute Australia); Dr Tony White (dermatologist); Dr Jo Matthews (cardiologist and inter- ventionalist); and Dr Ron Ehrlich (holistic dentist).

Thank you to my colleague and dear friend Teresa Mitchell- Paterson, I continue to learn from you constantly. Thank you for your time and proofreading in the book's early stages. Also to Rosemary Gillespie, director of Proof Communications, thank you for your tips and ongoing laughs, you are a treasure.

I would also like to thank Peter Sergeant from Mensheds Australia and Peter Williams for proofreading particular sections of the book.

Thank you to Australia's Prostate Foundation and the Bowel Cancer and Digestive Research Institute Australia for your warmth and generosity in giving me current information. I would also like to thank the Black Dog Institute and BeyondBlue for allowing me to use your well-researched facts. Thank you to the Cancer Council, Diabetes Australia and the Heart Foundation for your wonderful resources. These organisations help so many Aussies affected by the illnesses mentioned throughout the book and we need to support them in developing further research.

For those of you who were willing to share your story in this book for the benefit of other men, I thank you deeply. Thank you to Barry Daniels, Paul Scarfe and Russ Cooper and to those of you who preferred not to be identified.

I would like to thank both my work colleagues and dear friends for changing shifts to accommodate my work schedule, for listening to me processing my ideas, helping me stay focused and for your invaluable friendships. Special mention has to be given to Jim Ajouz, Fiona and Guy Donnellan, Belinda and Dave Roberts, Jules and Garry Davis, Lou Williamson, Kirsty Tilley, Sinead Davis, Libby and Nick Klein, Michelle Nosek, Natalie Haddrick, Leigh Killian, Helena Hewett, and to a man very dear to my heart, Neil Davidson. I cannot list everyone who has made an impact and shown such wonderful support, you know who you are so I thank you.

I hope you all enjoy this lighthearted yet informative read. Remember to stay healthy, stay informed!

www.ingramcontent.com/pod-product-compliance
Lightning Source LLC
Chambersburg PA
CBHW060028030426

42334CB00019B/2230